Senior Citizens Writing II

Senior Citizens Writing II

With an Introduction and Notes by
W. Ross Winterowd

Edited by
Bill Reid

Parlor Press
West Lafayette, Indiana
www.parlorpress.com

Parlor Press LLC, West Lafayette, Indiana 47906

Printed in the United States of America
S A N: 2 5 4 - 8 8 7 9

Library of Congress Cataloging-in-Publication Data

Senior citizens writing II / with an introduction and notes by
W. Ross Winterowd ; edited by Bill Reid.
    p. cm.
ISBN 978-1-60235-107-3 (pbk. : alk. paper) -- ISBN 978-1-
60235-108-0 (adobe ebook)
  1. Autobiographies--United States. 2. United States--
Biography. 3. Older people's writings, American. 4. Aging-
-Literary collections. I. Winterowd, W. Ross. II. Reid, Bill,
1930- III. Title: Senior citizens writng 2. IV. Title: Senior
citizens writing two.
CT101.S39 2009
808'.06692--dc22
                                    2009017701

Printed on acid-free paper.
Cover and book design by David Blakesley
Cover images ©
Thanks to Susan Bales for providing copy editing assistance on
this project.

Parlor Press, LLC is an independent publisher of scholarly
and trade titles in print and multimedia formats. This book is
available in paperback and Adobe eBook formats from Parlor
Press on the Internet at http://www.parlorpress.com. For sub-
mission information or to find out about Parlor Press publica-
tions, write to Parlor Press, 816 Robinson St., West Lafayette,
Indiana, 47906, or e-mail editor@parlorpress.com.

Preface

I thank Dr. W. Ross Winterowd for the encouragement, sage commentary, and friendship he so freely endowed on me, and generously endows on all older adult writing workshop attendees. I learned a great amount about life, writing, and story from his tireless efforts during the sixty workshop sessions I attended. I also attest that the many other workshop participants, who I now know as friends, have benefited in like manner, particularly the ten other authors who worked with me on the anthology section of this book.

Workshop attendees wish to thank the Huntington Beach Union High School and staff for their support for the Writing Workshops for older adults, sponsored since the Fall of 1999 and offered three times per year. We thank in particular Dr. Doris Longmead, principal of the Coast High School and Adult School, and her able staff; Catherine McGough, assistant principal at the school, and Dr. Winterowd's boss; Lynn Bergman, secretary; June Stark-Karaba, specialist for older adult classes; and Georgina Amparan, department secretary.

The patience and support of the anthology section authors was greatly appreciated, and I thank Paul Larkin, Joanne Simpson, and Marie Thompson for their reading, editing, and proofreading assistance on some of the contributions.

Thank you David Blakesley and Parlor Press for authorizing this second book on *Senior Citizens Writing*.

I give special thanks to Norma Winterowd and Tessa Reid, beloved wives whom Ross and I owe for the time we invested in the preparation of this book.

—Bill Reid

Acknowledgments

We are grateful for permission to reprint or adapt from the following sources:

Marjory Bong-Ray Liu: China map and inset: Courtesy of the University of Texas Libraries. The University of Texas at Austin. Excerpts included in "My Adventures in China During World War II" appeared in *Emeritus Voices*, the publication of the Arizona State University Emeritus College. Used by permission.

Richard Wrate: Excerpts from *The Aspen Times*: Courtesy of The Aspen Times, Inc.

Paul Larkin: "Ole George" and "The Paper Boy." Courtesy of *TomBigbee Country Magazine*.

Contents

Contents

Senior Citizens Writing II

Introduction

W. Ross Winterowd

You and I are exactly alike, you know. We both have limited time on this Earth, and we should choose to squeeze from the hours and days every possible drop of joy, every moment of peace. Even in this bleak age, with an even grimmer future. Of course, what I'm saying now makes perfectly good sense, but that sense is worthless. It adds up like two and two are four. Except that our adding machine is haywire, and good sense sometimes doesn't make sense. That's why all of us should lose ourselves in immensity. For every waking moment, we should try to make ourselves a part of eternity, that universe out there. When I was a boy, in summer I slept out on our back lawn, and I can remember gazing at the starry heavens and thinking that God must be there somewhere among the galaxies. Maybe when I was a boy I understood more than I do now. No one can know the infinite like you know the multiplication tables, but you can know it in your heart and soul, the joyous mystery of the whole thing. People used to talk about the music of the spheres. I think that I heard that music, more grand than any organ or choir. We all should try to hear that music again.

In groups of fifteen or so senior citizens huddle together, listening for a chord or a strain or a passage, and it's surprising how often we hear it. When we read Anna's story of the ramshackle house her father built, with varmints and bugs rustling in the walls; or the story of Michelle's doll that never smiled; or Art's tale about his wife's hats; or Paul's account of first sensing the awe and mystery of monastic life; or Phan's story about two lovers in wartime Viet Nam. . . . We perk up when we encounter the dissonance of Gerry's political tracts or the precision of Gordon's explanations of technology.

The term "creative writing" is anathema to us, for we believe that all serious writing is creative. Every well-crafted piece gives us echoes from the music of the spheres, those symphonies that we all heard when we were youngsters.

In our association with one another, in our work, and in our responses to that work, we find a mellow, autumnal music that is more satisfying than the rollicking melodies of spring or the songs of summer—because, of course, we know that the dirges of winter lie ahead.

Ah then, how do such marvels come about?

Here's the secret: people who want to write get together every week to read and respond to each other's work. That's such an arcane, mysterious concept, that I'll repeat it: people who want to write get together every week to read and respond to each other's work.

Years ago, a well-known scholar, one of my colleagues in the English Department at the University of Southern California, sputtered, "But everyone, ahem, knows, ahem, that you can't teach anyone to write." He was perfectly correct: you can't teach anyone to write or to play the cello or cast flies for trout—if by teaching you mean lecturing. But, of course, Piatagorsky would not have given a student a fifty-minute lecture on playing the cello (with the purpose of enabling the student to play the instrument), nor would Lee Wolf have given me a fifty-minute lecture on fly-casting. Both masters would probably have demonstrated first, then asked the student to attempt the passage or cast, and finally would have given feedback regarding the performance.

It is axiomatic, then, that the workshop leader be a writer, preferably a compulsive writer, who week-by-week shares his work with his workshop pals. (I have submitted sections of two novels, a couple of short stories, several essays on language and others on religion, as well as my series of vegetable poems, such as this one:

> Ah, parsnip, pallid winter root,
> Thou symbol, yes, that very fruit
> Of fallow fields and frozen ways,
> I alone will sing thy praise
> Before I whack thee quite in two
> And pop thee in this evening's stew.
> Oh, vegetable melancholic,
> When people dine and drink and frolic,
> Thou liest in the basement bin,
> A beetle bumbling blind therein.
> Thou suffer'st yet the worst of taunts:
> You're never served in restaurants.

The wonderful thing about the workshop is that all the participants very quickly become masters, able to give meaningful feedback to their colleagues. "I don't understand what you mean here. Can you clarify?" "You need more detail. I want to be able to 'see' that living room that's so important in your story." "Gee, you've bogged me down in too much detail. Why don't you cut some of it and get on with your story?" "I don't see how this paragraph relates to your whole purpose in this essay." "This sentence is hard to read. Can you rewrite so that it's more readable?"

A few rubrics are helpful, and as workshop leader, I slip them into our discussions. For instance: Four questions help writers with revision. "What can I *add* to make my story (essay, memoir) more interesting and credible?" "What should I *delete?*" "What can I *substitute* for this word (sentence, paragraph, image)?" "How can I *rearrange* to make this piece more convincing?"

We don't do any in-session writing. And we don't do much reading aloud. I know that many workshop leaders insist on "in-class" writing and that many also spend much of the time in sessions with participants reading their work aloud to the others. I know (and have written about) the mystique of "voice," a concept that I've never been really able to understand. I know a lot about style (syntax, usage, figures), arrangement, the adjustment of style and form for various audiences, the integrity (believability) of the writing, but I don't understand "voice." In other words, I can comment on syntax, diction, figures, development, and so on, but I don't know what I could say about voice. "Your voice in this story isn't authentic"? "Your voice in this essay is convincing"? "I really don't know what remarks such as that mean."

It's a hard and fast rule that any response to a piece of writing must be specific. "This is interesting" just doesn't cut it. We all want the "because."

Of course, writing of any genre is in bounds—except poetry. Participants are free to submit poetry, but I won't comment on poems. Most of the poetry that I have received through the years has been, I'm sure, heartfelt—but uninteresting as poetry. All of us are able to provide constructive feedback regarding fiction, memoirs, persuasive essays, and writings in other prose genres, but we're at a loss for useful feedback on poems. The poetry that workshop writers produce has, in my experience, almost inevitably been gushing in rhyme.

For the nuts and bolts about organizing and conducting writing workshops, I refer you to the long introduction to *Senior Citizens Writing* (Parlor Press, 2007).

Evaluating the success of a workshop is easy. If during the sessions there is much talk about the writing and a good deal of laughter, if the participants bond and become friends, if at the end of the ten- or twelve-week session the participants want to join the next session, if the workshop leader enjoys every minute of each session and cherishes his or her relationships with the participants—then the workshop has been a success.

Eddie Hasson

The lives that we in the workshop lived with Eddie were his three years as a submariner and his decades as a teacher. The selections that follow capture his enthusiasm and ebullience. Among the motives that bring senior citizens to the writing workshops are the desire to share their lives with others and to do that sharing in writing. After all, our meetings could have been bull sessions in which we exchanged anecdotes about our adventures and misadventures, but writing is a craft, and every craft gives its practitioners great opportunities for expression within the strictures that define the craft. The main opportunity and the main stricture regard audience. A personal letter to a close friend results from a set of tacit "rules" that would make an essay for strangers less than comprehensible. Chaim Perelman talked about "the universal audience." One goal of the workshop participants was to write for that universal audience, not simply for a good friend or close relative.

—W.R.W.

The Most Dynamic Class in Junior High School

In 1965, the Long Beach school system included a new class for seventh graders. It was a required one-semester class on coed health. Prior to that year, health was taught to seventh graders as a two week unit within their physical education class: boys by their men's P.E. teacher, girls by their women's P.E. teacher.

The new semester course for seventh graders included many more subjects: Growth and Development, Personal Health, Disease, Individual Changes during Puberty, Human Re-production, Male and Female reproductive systems, Family composition and Relationships. Also included were the usual subjects that were taught in the prior P.E. units: Mood-Modifiers, Drug Abuse, Alcohol and Tobacco, and First Aid. All the teachers who were to teach the Health classes took a special course at Long Beach State College. A teacher who had been teaching the class at a different school district taught it. This very valuable class was to prepare us for the teaching of subjects that would make seventh grade squirrels squirm.

I found that the actual day-to-day teaching of the various units would cause many other subject to arise. Questions would be asked. You could see the light turn on in the students faces'. "I didn't know that, Wow!"

Health class became the most dynamic class in school. Math class teaches math! History teaches history! Health classes . . . Wow!

Seventh graders run in age from approximately eleven and a half years to twelve and a half years, depending on when their parents started them in school. This age group is experiencing many changes, both mentally and physically—puberty. Some of the students are developing into young girls and young boys. While some of the same age students are still little *puppies.*

With every new class, my goal was to establish a rapport that would make the students comfortable in the subjects that were covered. They were told that they were allowed to ask questions at almost any point in our discussions. There were to be no written questions. Raise your hand and ask. Use proper words and phrases. During the unit on Human Reproduction, I would list both the male and female reproductive organs on one corner of the blackboard and leave it there during the entire unit. "I don't want to hear the words you might have picked up from a public bathroom wall, or from an off-color joke." Some students would look down at their desks or try to suppress a smile . . . Sneaky little kids!

"We will use a text book during this class. The most important part of this course is *class discussion,* I want each of you to participate in our discussions. I will call on you from time to time. Be ready. Oh, by the way, you will not be notified as to when there will be a test. The test will come a week or more after the unit is over. We will be in a new unit when, BANG, children, we have a test today! Do not panic, all of you were in on our discussions. Don't panic! The system works very well!"

In the first week, I wanted my students to know the meaning of two words. The first was *hypothetical.* I explained the meaning and told them we would be using hypothetical situations often in our discussions. The other word they were to know was *inhibitions.* That word would be important when discussing Alcohol and Drug Abuse. In all the years I taught Health, only once did a student know the definition of inhibitions, and none had heard of mood modifiers.

Our first unit was about mood modifiers. Of these eleven and twelve year old students, probably 100 percent had not been involved with drug abuse. Maybe a few had taken a puff or even smoked a whole cigarette and drank the remains of dad's drink or beer.

At this point I explain that the decision to enter into that kind of behavior is solely up to them. "*You decide.*" You don't ask Mom or Dad if you could smoke some *pot*. You know what the answer will be. Besides, they will get suspicious. "Who have you been hanging around with?" Dad asks, "What the hell is going on—go to your room, I want to talk to your Mom," etc.

Some students are nodding their heads in agreement. (No way!) I was often accused of sounding just like their dads. ("As long as you live in this house, you'll follow our rules!") If you ask your friends (peers) who are involved in that behavior, their answer will be. "No problem, I've been smoking grass for a long time. It's great, it's fun!" If you ask your older brother or sister, they will probably say, "You shouldn't, you're too young." Then they'll talk to Mom and Dad. "You better keep an eye on Jimmy. He asked me about smoking grass. I told him to stay away from the kids he's running around with. Some are really *screwed up.*"

"So you should make those decisions your self. You alone! In this class you will learn about the things that can happen if you become a smoker. How the excess drinking of alcohol can lower inhibitions, reduces reaction time. How doing drugs can alter your lives, becoming addicted. You will hear of many examples of successful people who get caught up in the drug scene and eventually ruined their careers and lives."

"Each of you is the most important person in your life. You are number one. Not Mom, not Dad. No one is more important than you! So, after knowing the results of smoking, drinking, and drug abuse, you will sit in your room all alone, and make decisions about your life. Not all at once."

"Do I want to do this to myself? Do I want to please my peers or lose them? If I don't smoke *pot* they probably don't want me around. What should I do? Can I get new friends?" As seventh graders they all state that "I'm not going to get involved."

I tell them "I will know if I've been a successful teacher if I can *quiz* you ten or fifteen years from now to see how each of you are getting along in your lives. Be strong. You are Number One."

I taught one class of Health and four classes of Physical Education per semester, for many years—I actually got paid for it!

I got a backhanded compliment from our counselor. She pretended to complain that she had to change certain students programs after a parent phone call: "My oldest daughter had Mr. Hasson for Health. I want my seventh grade daughter to be in Mr. Hasson's class."

It made me feel that I was doing a good job of teaching Health. I was very pleased.

Human Reproduction

The most rewarding subject in teaching the seventh grade co-ed Health Class, is Human Reproduction. It is rewarding to the teacher to see the students getting information about something they know something about, but are not sure if they've got it right. A few of them have been told by one or both of their parents, a few are not sure because they got *bits and pieces* from their peers, older friends or from hearing *off color jokes.* On such subjects, in many cases, they confess they are reluctant to ask questions, even to parents. At the start of the unit, there is a tendency on the part of the students to be *walking on eggshells!* In many cases, they are not familiar with the vocabulary of the male and female reproductive organs. They definitely are uncomfortable in listening to or discussing sexual intercourse!

My job first was to make the class comfortable with the subject, and to use proper words in our discussions. As I've mentioned in previous papers, I would write on the blackboard the proper names of the male and female reproductive organs and leave them there during the entire two-week unit. The class was given a booklet on the subject to study. The major part of the class was discussion.

My opening statement was "Everyone in this class including the teacher, has a belly button. If there is anyone in this class who does not have a belly button, he or she must be from Mars!"

That would set the stage for the first day. The fact that we were all born was because of a mother and father's union. The first thing in our discussion was about the umbilical cord. In beginning with that subject, the students started thinking and asking questions.

At all times I used the expression "When a husband and wife decide to have children." Little by little, the students felt more comfortable with the subject.

One of the more interesting reactions was when we talked about when females began to menstruate. I explained that girls around their age start having their period at different times, not all exactly at the same age. It varies with each person. Also, that normally females menstruate approximately every four weeks between puberty and menopause. What most of the students didn't know, and were very surprised to hear, was that a rich layer of blood formed on the walls of the uterus every four weeks in preparation for receiving a fertilized ovum (egg cell), so that it will develop into a baby.

Shock! "Mr. Hasson, do you mean once a month this happens?"

"Yes, and when there is no fertilized egg, the body gets rid of the blood. That is what menstruation is all about!" The girls knew something about menstruation; very few knew the reason for their monthly period.

When I told them that when a wife missed her period, there was a possibility that she was pregnant. You could see their minds processing this information. Hands were raised, questions asked! No time to be timid! Stories about moms missing her period, a false alarm! These seventh graders wanted to know more!

Co-Ed Health—Undivided Attention

When the subject of Sexual Intercourse was discussed, I had the complete attention of the class. Everyone alert. Every ear was tuned in, although many eyes were looking down at their desks. (In all the years that I taught Health, only two or three families had their child excused from that particular unit.)

I started with when a husband and wife love each other and decide to start a family, they have sexual intercourse. Sexual intercourse is usually done in bed, that the man is usually on top, etc. (All through the discussion, I keep an eye on the class members to see if they are coping with the subject.) The words *penis, vagina,* and *sperm,* are used. When the explanation is over, there are very few questions. Much thinking. On the days following, there are many questions. Always, the question, "Do you only have sexual intercourse if you want children?"

"No, a married couple love each other and enjoy sex. It is a very intimate showing of how much they love each other."

In one class, a boy asked, "Do you have to go to a hospital when you have sexual intercourse?" He was completely serious.

On the following days, we talk about pregnancy, the changes in the mother that take place in the nine months, give or take, for the baby to be born. When it's close to the birth time, mom and dad will make a dry run to the hospital. That is to make sure they know where to go and park when it is time. Things can get hectic, and time saved can be important. Mom packs a suitcase with things she will need at the hospital and has it ready. When the labor pains start, there is no time to waste!

One time I was explaining about labor pains. "When the baby is about to be born, it will be in a head down position in the uterus."

A girl in the front row raised her hand. "Mr. Hasson, Mr. Hasson."

"Yes, Laura, what is it?"

"When I was born I was a butt first baby." Out of the mouths of babes! I started to laugh . . . I had to hold on to my desk. (The class loved it when they would say something to make me laugh—which was often.)

"Now Laura, how did you know that?"

"My mom told me." I knew her mom, and later she confirmed the story.

During the explanation of male sperm cells and female ovum (egg cells), I stated that the male sperm cell determined the sex of the newborn—boy or girl. I was continuing on the subject and heard someone talking near the back of the room. I stopped and saw that it was Nancy P. She wasn't talking to anyone in particular, she was actually *grumbling* to herself. "Nancy, what seems to be the problem?"

"Mr. Hasson, you just said the male sperm determines the sex of the baby!"

"That's right, Nancy."

"Well, I just saw the movie about King Henry VIII this weekend. Two of his wives, Anne Boleyn and Catherine of Aragon, gave birth to girls, not boys, so he had them put to death. It was *his* fault, not theirs." Nancy was furious! I explained that in those days, medical science didn't know about sperm and ovum. They didn't know about chromosomes and genes. Nancy couldn't be placated. (I loved those kids.)

We talked about the unfortunate situations like *stillborn* or *miscarriage*, when a woman had to visit her gynecologist to have a D&C. "Mr. Hasson. Mr. Hasson," hand waving frantically in the air. (This was the usual reaction when a student, usually a girl, knew the answer.)

"Yes, Leslie, what is it?"

"I know what a D&C is."

"Tell us!"

"My mom said it's "Dusting and Cleaning.""

How can you not love the enthusiasm and spontaneity of that age group?

These are just some of the many great moments in teaching Co-Ed Health to seventh graders.

First Aid Unit

Surprisingly, seventh graders were very interested in the two week First Aid unit. Starting with the definition of First Aid: The Immediate and temporary care given a victim of an accident or sudden illness until the services of a physician can be obtained. We covered wounds, severe bleeding, injuries to bones, joints, and muscles, poison by mouth, burns, and artificial respiration.

It was interesting and amusing hearing from the students as to how they convinced their parents to put together a First Aid Kit for the house or the family car. In class, we practiced with bandages, splints, triangular bandages, and discussed how to carry victims and when not to move them.

When we came to First Aid for a drowning victim, I would demonstrate the *back pressure arm lift* method. We then discussed the method using *mouth-to-mouth* to resuscitate a victim. That it was the best method of artificial respiration . . . clear victims mouth of any foreign matter . . . tilt head back . . . chin pointing upward . . . open your mouth wide . . . place tightly over victim's mouth . . . pinch victim's nostril's shut. For an adult, blow vigorously about 12 breaths per minute . . . For a child, take relatively shallow breaths at the rate of 20 per minute.

"Okay, students, tomorrow we will practice the mouth-to-mouth method of artificial respiration. You will practice on each other! So pick a partner. Boys ask girls—girls ask boys—or girl a girl, or boy a boy. In any case, have a partner. If not, I will pair you up! This will be a big part of your grade. If you are absent, you will practice when you return." There was stunned silence! Students looking down at their desks. Some boys grinning, some boys terrified! Most students in a panic mode! (Hasson, you're mean!)

The next day, the class came in quietly. Not a peep! I took role, then reminded them that we were to practice the mouth-to-mouth method of artificial respiration. "It is important that you learn this. Who knows when you might be called on to save a little boy or girl, or your mother or father." Quiet throughout the class.

"Oh, by the way, class. I want to introduce you to a friend of mine." The class looks up . . . what is he talking about? I bring up from behind my desk, a suitcase. I set it on the long table and open it. "I want you to meet *Resusci-Anne.*" I pulled out this dummy that is provided by the Red Cross. It is used to practice the mouth-to-mouth method. She has a plastic face, arms and legs. You blow into her mouth, her chest rises and falls. The class explodes . . ."Mr. Hasson, you are so mean . . . I couldn't sleep last night . . . I didn't want to come to school today, my mother made me." Smiles and chuckles . . . Everyone gathered around the table and took turns practicing on *Annie.* I would wipe her mouth with alcohol each time and the next student would give it a try. The lesson went very well, it was a good learning experience, with many laughs. I hoped that the lesson would come in handy in the future of those students—students who are now adults, and probably married, with children of their own.

Coed Health Class House Rules

I ask the question, "What are the rules at your house about keeping your room neat and clean?" Whenever we discuss subjects about the home and family, the students are interested to hear about other households. Freddie raises his hand. "What's your story, Freddie?"

"My mom says that it's my room and if I want to live in a *pig pen,* that's my problem. Just keep it in my room."

The other students voice surprise and amazement. "Man, he's lucky!" Stories abound as to rules at different households.

Hands go up all over the room. "My mother has inspection of my room every Saturday. I can't do anything until my room passes inspection: hang clothes in closet, shoes on closet floor neatly! Games, books, etc, must be stored in their proper places. Actually, I'm glad she makes me do that once a week. Sometimes I fool her, and have my room clean before she comes in. That's because I've got something to do on Saturday that I don't want to miss."

Pam states that her mom checks her room anytime she wants. It better be neat! Everything must be in its proper place at all times. Wow!

Jennifer had the wildest story about *house rules.* "My mother . . ." (there was never a story about Dad being involved in the room being clean and neat. Very interesting?) "My mother can't stand to have things left on the table in the hall that is just inside the front door. I leave my jacket and books on the table. My brother drops his stuff on the table. My dad comes home. He takes off his coat and leaves it on the table along with a folder or whatever else he brings home. My mother has told us not to clutter up the day table! She has a big wooden box in the back yard. She picks up whatever is on the table, takes it outside and throws it into the box—no matter what it is or who owns it! The box has no cover. If it's raining—too bad! If you don't want it in the box, put it away, not on the table. Sometimes

we're in a hurry . . . gotta use the bathroom . . . fast!
Then we forget to pick up our stuff—too bad!"

Jennifer told us that one time her dad put his stuff
down on the table. Mom threw it all into the box. Later
he was going to give Mom her birthday present. He
went to the hall table to get it. Not there! Hey, rules are
rules! Different rules at different houses!

A Sad Story

After teaching three years at Stephens, a brand new ju-
nior high was built, Marshall Junior High School. Our
principal was to transfer there, so he asked a few of his
staff if we would like to go with him. He wanted me to
be head of the P.E. department. I jumped at the chance
and spent six wonderful years there. There were many
highlights, and, of course, a few sad situations. This
happened in 1956, before coed P. E.

The teacher's lounge, where most teachers ate lunch,
was across campus. Bernice J., one of the Home Eco-
nomics teachers, volunteered her room so that we could
eat lunch to avoid the long trek. We were brown bag-
ging, so it worked out well. About six or eight teachers
took advantage of the offer. These teachers were good
friends and each had a good sense of humor. Lunch
was fun!

One day we walked in for lunch and sat around our
usual table. Over at the other end of the room sat a
ninth grade girl eating her lunch. Two of the teachers
had her in class. They called to her "Hi, Janice." She
smiled and gave a little wave. The fact that a student

was in the room put a cramp in our conversation. No joking around. Be nice, Ed!

Near the end of the lunch period, Bernice told the girl to go on to her next class. As soon as she left, we asked Bernie, what had she done to have to spend her lunch period in the room? Bernie explained that she wasn't being punished, but had asked if she could eat in the room. She had been gaining weight and some of the kids were teasing her at lunch, and she was embarrassed. (Junior high kids can be the cruelest.) We all felt sorry for her, but also felt restricted in our conversation. Bernie said, "I know, I'll talk with her."

The next day *it* hit the fan. Bernie called Janice in during her conference period. Early in the talk, Janice started to cry. She broke down and stated that she didn't know who to turn to. She was pregnant! She didn't know what to do, and was hysterical as Bernie tried to console her

The girl was not popular in school. She had few friends, was rather shy, and mostly kept to herself. She was terrified about telling her mother. It turned out that her mother worked nights. Bernie asked her, "Did you go out with your boy friend at night, and your mother doesn't know about it?" Janice screamed through her tears, "I don't have a boy friend. It was my stepfather!"

Ms. J. told Janice she would go with her to see the girls' vice principal, that the V.P. would help her, and that the district had a school with a class for pregnant students. Also, she would call her mother for a conference and then let her know the situation. It would be easier that way. "Janice, you can't face this alone."

In the vice principal's office, Mrs. H., a former P. E. teacher, was just the right person for this situation. She was kind and understanding (she could also be tough when the situation warranted it).

Janice was told that a school psychologist would counsel her, and that Mrs. H. would have her mother come in for a conference. At that time, she would let her mother know the situation.

Two days later, Janice's mother came to school. Because she worked nights, it was no trouble to meet with the vice principal. First, Mrs. H. wanted to meet with Janice's mother alone. She was told, in a very patient way, that her daughter was pregnant. A shock! She got up and walked back and forth in the small office. She finally sat down. "I didn't even know she went out with boys, or that she had a boy friend!"

Janice was then brought into the office, and was already crying. Mom stood up and took her daughter in her arms and, soon, both were crying. Janice finally settled down. Her mother asked Janice if she had been going out at night, if she had a boy friend, and if so, who was it? Janice looked at her mother and stammered, "It was Bill. I don't go out at night. I don't have a boy friend." She screamed, "It was Bill!" She bent over, crying.

Mom could not believe what she was hearing. "You mean, it was your step father . . ."

Janice didn't look up, "Yes," she said quietly. After a few moments, Mrs. H. took Janice to the nurse's office to lie down. Mom sat quietly, just staring.

Mom looked up. "Can I use your phone?" Mrs. H. pushed the phone over to her. She called the police, and while waiting for the connection, she looked up. "My husband is outside, waiting in the car. He drove me here."

In about ten minutes, two police officers walked into the vice principal's office, and were told what the situation was by Janice's mother. Mrs. H. told them the rest of the story. The police got a description and were told that the stepfather was outside waiting in the car.

The two officers walked out and approached him. They asked the stepfather to step out of the car. He was handcuffed, put into the police car, and taken to the station.

This happened in 1956. Our entire faculty was devastated. Janice was checked out of our school, and sent to live with a relative. We never knew what happened with Janice's mom or the stepfather or even if she had the baby.

On occasion, some of our students go through hell. Some try to get through it alone. How sad.

Talent Shows and Other Performances at the Junior High Level

A junior high school stage performance is always outstanding. There is no such thing as a flop. The very fact that the talent is made up of amateurs makes the show acceptable. Even when lines are forgotten or other mistakes occur, it's part of what makes it memorable.

The school orchestra or band is playing a popular melody or a classic composition. The Glee Club is performing in the annual Christmas show or in a musical assembly. No matter, you watch and listen with a smile on your face, or at times, a tear running down your cheek.

If it's an evening performance, it's a packed house. Every parent is there to watch their *little darlings* take their first step toward an entertainment career. Parents enjoy the entire show, but the focus is primarily on their child. Not so with the teacher, especially this Physical Education teacher. I would be constantly surprised to see my students in a completely different role!

There on stage is Robert L., who in my class can be heard the minute he walks into the locker room, yelling at a friend or teasing someone. Sometimes it's me. He has his motor running the entire P. E. period. On stage, Robert is standing in the tenor section of the chorus. He is wearing a white shirt a black tie (mom tied it for him, I'm sure.) He is quiet—looking only at his teacher. He has an *angelic* look on his face. When the chorus starts to sing, they all look like angels. What a beautiful sound!

I spot other students who are in my classes. Unbelievable. At another assembly, the orchestra is playing. I stare and smile. Ralph R., my defensive lineman on our Saturday League football team, is playing the kettledrums. He has that serious look you often see on kettledrummers.

On one occasion at an evening show, Ken T., the orchestra teacher, was about to lead his students. He tapped the podium for attention. He raised the baton and the orchestra started to play, but something didn't sound right to him. He tapped several times on the podium, and said something to the orchestra. They stopped playing . . . they looked stunned. I'm sure I could see smoke coming out of Ken's ears! He tapped again, raised his baton, and the orchestra had never sounded better. At the finish, the audience gave them a standing ovation. Junior high school kids never cease to amaze.

Old Mother Hubbard

At Stephens Junior High, in 1953, we were going to have a Talent Show. I had been teaching gymnastics to a group of students. They had been playing football, baseball, and running most of their young lives— gymnastics was a new activity for them. A few found a real love for the sport, but not all students jumped on the bandwagon. Those that did couldn't get enough of horizontal bars, parallel bars, tumbling, and long-horse vaulting.

On the gym team, I had a group of small but strong seventh graders who became very good tumblers. I wondered about having them perform in the talent show. I talked to our art teacher, Phyllis B., about these boys. After I described what they did as tumblers, Phyllis suggested they play the children of the "Old lady who lived in a shoe." Phyllis volunteered to make the prop, a very large shoe with windows that the tumblers could dive-roll out of.

It was a smash hit! The curtain opened, and there was this great big shoe. It had a smoke stack at the top, shoestrings painted all the way down, and two large windows with painted curtains. I had a row of tumbling mats on the floor in front of the shoe.

It was completely quiet. An off stage voice came on: "There was an old lady who lived in a shoe. She had so many children she didn't no what to do." There was silence . . . Then one after another, the tumblers came diving out through the windows, and ran to one end of the mats. They were in their glory! Round-off back handsprings, front handsprings, front flips, back flips, then their own combinations of stunts. In all, they each had four runs. Then one after another they dive-rolled back through the windows (mats were placed on the other side, also—I'm not a cruel person.) It was again very quiet . . . Then curtains closed to loud applause, and hoopin' and hollerin'!

We probably could have taken that show on the road. Broadway?

Mary Ann Huisken

The workshop participants are, after all, senior citizens—some of us very senior. Many of the pieces that come out of the workshop are documents that record the history and mores of a past generation, pre-TV, even pre-talking movies. Edna Woolley tells of seeing and hearing the first talkie, "The Jazz Singer"; Marjory Liu gives us a virtual "documentary" on life in China during the Japanese occupation; Paul Larkin's tales of life in a Mississippi town during the 1930s are in the tradition of Jacob Riis. Mary Ann's vivid account of life on her grandparents' farm and of decorating the Christmas tree are warm and colorful, but also valuable as cultural documents.

One of the maxims that we stress again and again in the workshops is the necessity for seemingly insignificant details (borrowing from G. K. Chesterton, I call them "tremendous trifles") that, one after another, bring the writing to life—for example, Mary Ann's information about the time zones and their significance for the family or the menus for dinner and supper.

—W.R.W.

A City Girl on the Farm

Annual June to September summer trips to my grandparent's farm in Danville, Illinois, were the highlights of my life. In California, I lived a somewhat quiet life, as an only child with both parents working, coming straight home from school doing homework and some chores, then waiting for my dad to get home at 5:30 p.m.—it was a nice life, but lonely at times. When at my grandparent's farm, with people around all the time, there was never a lack of things to do, animals to enjoy, and cousins to play with.

The farm was uniquely located on the Illinois/Indiana state line, which was also a time zone change. One hundred twenty acres on the Indiana side went by Eastern Time, while their home and another hundred and thirty acres were in Illinois, operating an hour earlier on Central Time. Scheduling family functions was always followed by the clarification of whether it was Illinois or Indiana time.

There were shops in downtown Danville, but my time on the farm was spent playing with cousins who lived nearby, mostly helping my grandparents in any way I could. Sundays were our day to dress up and go to church, and afterwards have dinner with the family at one of their homes. Once or twice during my stay, I'd go to the local drive-in-movie with my older cousins, or to the skating rink with my cousin, Kay. There was no television at the farm, but we did listen to the radio for the most important news of the day— the weather predictions, and sometimes at night we'd all gathered to enjoy a radio program.

Grandma could usually be found in the kitchen, preparing meals for Grandpa and the other field helpers. Sometimes a dozen people would appear at the noon hour, which they called "dinner," each of them tired and hungry. Although they were poor, Grandma prepared filling meals; dinner was the main meal of the day, and usually included chicken, homemade noodles, cottage cheese, sliced red ripe tomatoes, vegetables from the garden, and occasionally meat. I loved the wonderful creamed peas and new potatoes, which were both home grown. Everything tasted so good. The evening meal, called "supper," was light compared to dinner, and often was what they called "milk toast," browned buttered toast torn in pieces, put in a tall glass and covered with warm sweetened milk. It wasn't much, but it was delicious and filled our tummies for the night.

Grandpa was a tall, emaciated looking man, with a leathery looking face, tanned from long days in the sun. He always wore the same gray striped coveralls, and a cap that was often cocked, covering his straight gray hair. He'd come in from the fields looking like he was near dead from exhaustion. Usually, he would wash his hands in a bucket of wash water, sit down, briskly rub his aching knees, tell about his days activities, then eat with all who were there. Many days, as Grandpa returned to the fields after dinner, he would let two or three of us grandchildren ride down the lane with him on his International M-tractor, as we stood on the wheel wells, hanging on tightly to him, or sitting in his lap. Sometimes he would put his hand over ours and let us crank the gears a little—what a thrill that was. At times, he would be pulling a 10–12 foot wide disc or a three-bottom plow. Looking back, I'm amazed that none of us fell and got hurt—when our grandparents told us to do something, like hang on—we did it!

There was never a lack of things to do, according to our Grandma, who was short, heavy, had a head full of graying red hair, and had the personality to go with it. She had large round hazel eyes that got your attention and she was the one we ran to when hurt or needing a hug. She was the taskmaster, a hard worker, and a wonderful cook. All summer long, Grandma directed us to areas on the farm that needed attention. She told us how to do things, but didn't micro manage or yell at us when we did it wrong. One time I took my turn at mowing their large yard and mowed down the center of her prized rose garden; no one had told me how to turn off the mower, and I couldn't make it turn. I knew those roses were very special to her and I cried my eyes out over my mistake. The next spring she wrote a letter to me, telling me how healthy her roses were coming up after my "summer pruning." That was Grandma. She yelled at us, but rarely got mad. She often sent us kids out to her large vegetable gardens to weed, pull carrots or onions, dig potatoes, pick peas, green beans, and tomatoes from the vines. But our favorite chore was picking sweet corn, because we made a game of running and hiding in the rows of corn before picking it and bringing it in.

One of our special rewards for helping Grandma was being able to go into the fenced-in chicken yard to play in the old apple tree. We cousins would run through the chicken yard, scattering hens every direction to get to the apple tree that grew near the highway on the north side of the farm. The tree was old and had huge sprawling branches that supported all of us kids; it was better than any man-made toy and was perfect for our fantasy play. Any brave chickens that roamed under the tree branches were in enemy territory, ours, and although we never hurt any of them, we defended our positions in the tree branches with fierce verbal shooting sounds, and by dropping leaves and bird-pecked rotten green apples to the ground. The chickens clucked and flew away. Slowly they would return to see if there might be any juicy wiggling worms left in the apples, and our games continued. Oh, how we loved playing in that tree, climbing from one limb to another, trading limb positions with each other, depending who wanted to be highest, next to someone specific, or further out on a limb. Our days passed quickly and happily. One summer lightning struck the apple tree and split it in half. We were all devastated at that loss, but switched to playing in the hayloft in the barn— complete with mice, bugs, and our favorite farm cats.

As far back as I can remember, Grandma and Grandpa would take me into the chicken yard on the side of the house and let me hold the tiny baby yellow chicks. Handling them gently was a requirement and putting them back near their nest was, too. Grandma's tattered blue apron had large pockets that she filled with feed when we went to see the chicks. She'd hold her hand out steady until a chicken spotted the food and came over to eat, then Grandpa would support my hand and move it closer to Grandma's until it was close enough for her to put some feed in mine, encouraging me not to be afraid, or to move. The chickens slowly approached and pecked feed from my hand, and it wasn't long until I was brave enough to hold my hand out alone. It seemed to me the chickens wasted as much of the feed as they ate; they were messy. And if they ate one bite, they pooped two.

Grandma often sent me out to the chicken pen with a little basket to collect eggs, and I was careful not to break any before getting them back to the house. I knew to enter the coops slowly so I wouldn't scatter the hens and have them clucking at me. Hens didn't need contact with roosters to lay eggs, but needed them to lay fertilized eggs and have baby chicks. Most of the hens were content to just lay regular eating eggs. The laying hens sat on their nests all day long, laying an egg a day, and they would generally let me move them a little to stick my hand under them to collect the eggs they were sitting on. Once in a while, a rooster would come around when I was there, and some were mean; they would come right up to me, shaking their floppy red combs and peck me with their pointed beaks, letting me know it was time for me to go.

One day when none of my cousins were there to play and I was getting a little bored, Grandma said, "Why don't you go out and collect some eggs for me?" Well, that sounded like a good idea and I took my basket and went out to the chicken yard. I collected a few eggs from the smaller of the two chicken coops and then went to the larger one in the center of the yard, and thought: I'm really going to make Grandma happy, and collect every single egg in the yard, no matter how hard they are to get. After collecting eggs from the nests inside the coops, I noticed there were some different nests under the coop that was raised off the ground about ten inches. So, I got a stick, lay on the dirty ground, and using my stick, collected all the eggs I could see. It took me a while, and the chickens were not happy about me using the stick, but I was determined to get all of the eggs. I carried them to Grandma, pretty proud of myself for doing such a good job; she gave me a special hug and smile, and told me to put the eggs in the refrigerator. Grandma's voice was all I needed to be happy, though sometimes it was sort of mean sounding, like when yelling to get us kids to come in or do something. But we knew no matter how she yelled, she loved us.

The next morning, I was in the kitchen when Grandma was making breakfast for Grandpa. She was breaking eggs in the skillet and suddenly shrieked, "Ee-eech! . . . Oh no!"

"What, Grandma?" I asked. She looked over at me and said, "Sis, where did you collect eggs yesterday?" I told her I had done the best job I had ever done, collecting every egg in the yard and both chicken coops. She didn't say another word, just emptied the skillet with the un-hatched baby chick into the trash container, and went to get another egg out of the refrigerator, not knowing whether it would be an egg for eating, or a fertilized, baby chick egg collected by mistake. Grandma never scolded me, but my older cousins told me I had collected and ruined the baby chicken crop—I felt horrible about having done that. My grandparents were poor, and worked hard on the farm to earn money to survive and to let us grandchildren come to stay with them. And in my naiveté, I was solely responsible for destroying the baby chick crop. I thought about what to do, and told Grandma and Grandpa I was sorry; they made light of it and changed the subject to something fun.

Fairly regularly, Grandma and some of my aunts would prepare to "do chickens," as they would say. That's when we kids got to go on chicken hunts, with reshaped wire clothes hangers that had been stretched out straight except for one end that was hooked to catch chickens. We would all enter the chicken yard with our hooked wires; chase a chicken, swiping at it until we had it hooked by its feet. Then we'd run out the gate, the chicken squawking and dangling from our hooks, slam the chicken on the ground, and Grandma or one of our aunts would quickly step on the chicken's head, grab the feet and pull, separating the head from the body; the body would flop around the yard, splattering blood all over. Sometimes we'd look around and see headless chickens hopping in the yard, then we would run and scream "Eeee-yuk!", then go back into the chicken yard looking for another victim. It was quite a production line, and all of us had fun being part of it. Once the bodies stopped flopping around, Grandma would take them by the feet and drop them into a galvanized tub filled with hot water, to make it easier to pluck the feathers off the chicken's body. She called it "dressing the chicken," but to me, it always looked like they were being undressed. Each "do chickens" day, we accumulated quite a pile of chickens for Grandma. I didn't know until later in my life that Grandma sold these chickens to individuals in town who sometimes preordered 20–30 at a time.

One of the biggest changes for me from city to farm life was the outhouse. The outhouse was about twenty yards from the back porch, and it was dark at night while hot and fly infested during summer days. I had an unfounded fear that a snake or some other creature would crawl out of the hole while I was there using it. I'm sure that some of my older male cousins told me "stories" they swore were true regarding outhouse creatures. Usually, one of my girl cousin's and I went together; one to hold the door slightly open for light, and to be there in case the other accidentally fell in. Modesty wasn't even a thought. I was almost a teen when the old one-hole wooden outhouse was replaced with a newer one that had two holes for people to sit. For me, that was a great improvement, and I loved having one of my cousins go sit with me.

I was in junior high school when my grandparents finally got plumbing in the house. One of the bedroom closets in the house was converted to an indoor bathroom, with toilet, washbasin, and bathtub. At the same time, a small bedroom for guests and us grandkids was added just off the kitchen. There was much excitement that summer, and when all was finished, we thought that house was as up-to-date as one could get—all 900 square feet of it.

Compared to the city, sometimes farm life in the Midwest was very difficult because of the severe weather changes. Occasional tornados caused everyone to stop what they were doing, rush back to the fields, and do what they could to protect the crops.

I look back fondly to those days on the farm and am thankful for all of the things I learned from my grandparents, aunts, uncles and cousins that I never would have known from living in a city in sunny Southern California. The satisfaction of a job well done, crops sold for good prices, and helping one another as family or friends was the ultimate reward. Fortunately, I had this wonderful opportunity of learning much from my grandparents.

Sleeping Under the Stars

Before finishing my last year of college, I met and married another student named John, who had graduated with his bachelor's degree and was starting graduate school. We married during winter break, then went back to school, both taking full-time class loads so we could finish college as soon as possible. We had part time jobs at night, so come summer, we felt entitled to a vacation.

For some time John had been dropping hints about going on a back packing trip during the summer. Since that was months away, I chose to just let him talk about it, hoping some other idea would come up, one that would better suit both of us. But by spring, it was clear that this idea of camping out under the stars, tent-less, was more than just a passing thought. When we were around friends, some sort of discussion about hiking the John Muir trail through the Yosemite wilderness area up to Tuolumne Meadows always came up. One night while out with our best friends Dick and Elaine, who were also newlyweds, the two guys started discussing *our* summer trip to Yosemite when school was out. After a grueling semester of classes, homework, night jobs and now keeping house, my idea of a vacation was going somewhere to lie around the pool and sleep, not hike dusty trails, sleep on the ground in sleeping bags, cook over a camp stove, and walk miles each day. Every opportunity Elaine and I had to talk that evening, we shared our concerns and threw in our ideas of a good vacation, but they fell on deaf ears. Our husbands had decided on this back packing trip and were oblivious to our reluctance, and frankly, were too newly married and inexperienced to realize this was a disaster in the making. They spent the evening trying to get us excited about getting new hiking boots, backpacks, and going shopping for dehydrated food to cook. Near the end of the night, they made the mistake of asking us what we thought about our trip. It didn't take a minute for my response. I wished the two of them well and hoped they had a good time—I was not going and that was that! But it wasn't.

We started having nightly pillow chats about backpacking that were neither friendly nor conducive to good sleep. To top it off, my mother was outspoken in supporting my thoughts about this being a good trip for the guys, but not for me. John was furious at her. Our exchanges were unkind causing us to dress and leave for school without saying much to each other. I dreaded everything about the backpacking trip, except for being in the company of our friends. I wanted to be thought of as a good wife, so I finally agreed to go. My friend, Elaine, couldn't believe I said "yes," and wanted to strangle me. She had counted on my strength to say "no" for both of us, but she relented, too. We agreed to go, so our husbands would know we were supportive. Reluctantly, we got our own equipment, including lightweight sleeping bags, backpacks with racks, and boots that looked like U.S. Army issue. We also chose the freeze-dried foods, and were amazed at the variety available.

As it got closer to vacation time, on every walk I took to get used to my big clunky hiking boots, I thought, what have I done? The boots were ugly as well as heavy, and the only comfort I had in wearing them was that they would protect me from snakes I might step on. I am a true city girl, afraid of anything that slithers, creeps, crawls, or is bigger than me. My dreams about this trip were more like nightmares—encounters with snakes! John had done a lot of hiking while growing up and assured me he had never seen a snake, and said he would protect me from anything out there. He artfully embellished his comments with the blessings of camping outside in natural environments, and made me feel immature for suggesting there could ever be problems.

With college over for the spring semester, our vacation week had arrived—much too quickly. The guys carefully packed our gear in the car and were in vacation mood, ready for a grand adventure. We two girls were silently praying for a car breakdown, or anything else that would lend an opportunity to cancel this vacation, but we were glad to be together, and even looked forward to seeing Yosemite. Once we arrived and checked in with the rangers, the guys quickly unpacked the car, and double-checked they hadn't forgotten anything. Then without discussion, they shouldered most of the gear and took off towards the Tuolumne Meadows trail.

Day one hiking wasn't too bad. The trail to Tuolumne Meadows was easy and well used. We made good time considering this was our first time carrying all of our gear on our backs. The trail wound its way through open stretches, up steep rocky areas, across grassy meadows, and through forests of magnificent trees reaching high for the sunlight. The freshness and subtle pine fragrance was wonderful. John was right, darn him; I found the wilderness beautiful, and exciting to be in. Along the trail, we passed hikers coming down the trail, looking happy but dirty. My guess was they were anxious to get their boots off and have a shower. We stopped for the night at a cleared area in the woods. The guys were in their glory as they efficiently set up camp, then prepared dinner (part of our bargain). After a surprisingly good meal, they suggested that before dark, we use the outhouse a short distance from camp. Although I was excited about sleeping out under the stars, I didn't expect how very dark it got without city lights. That first night, each couple zipped our two sleeping bags together and I fell asleep as soon as I put my head down.

There were segments of this new adventure I absolutely loved. I felt completely liberated and free to get up and go without putting on makeup or fussing with my hair. The day two trek was a bit more difficult, with areas where we had to climb massive rock slopes, a challenge for me. My fear wasn't of falling, as much as it was reaching my hand up where a snake might strike it. But, once we got up onto the top, our husbands were so proud of us, their praises made it worth the effort. We had seen a few people on the trail that day, but not as many as the previous day. That evening, we felt like we were really away from civilization. Our macho husbands again prepared dinner, making it a memorable time. We got in our sleeping bags just as darkness took over. The guys pointed out various constellations in the sky, but all I really saw were millions of tiny, brilliant blinking stars. I was amazed how many stars there were. The four of us lay near each other, and for a few minutes talked about the interesting plants and blossoms we had seen along the trail then we playfully, noisily, took deep breaths of sparkling fresh air, before drifting into a deep sleep.

Day three was a challenge from the beginning. We did not see anyone all day, climbing and hiking steadily. The guys charged ahead, while we girls began to lag a little, and mumble under our breath as only girls can do, about this "wonderful trip." Elaine was a tall slender girl with shiny black hair, and she had a longer walking stride than me. We settled into our own pace, and I was clearly the slowest of all. Late in the afternoon, 50 feet behind the others, I was tired and feeling sorry I had agreed to come on this trip. My idea of fun wasn't hiking in the woods all day long with a heavy backpack pinching my shoulders. I really didn't like being behind everyone, so I decided to take a short cut across a green grassy area just off the trail, shortening the distance between all of us. I had taken about 15 steps when a large snake startled me as it quickly slithered away. I was shocked motionless, not only to see it, but how fast it moved. All my life I have been fearful of snakes, and this was the first real snake I had ever seen. My heart was pounding as adrenalin pumped through my body. My worst fear of the trip had just been realized. Snakes! A few steps later, another snake writhed in front of me. Two snakes! The rest of my steps were longer, higher, faster. I don't remember actually touching ground the rest of the way because I was so scared. I was still frantic when I caught up to the others, and began walking in their footprints. While setting up camp, all I could think about was snakes. In times of anger or fear I tend to clam up, I didn't say anything but my mind was screaming: *Yes, sweetheart—there are snakes here. Don't give me any of your "I've never seen any snakes," because I've seen two of them: today!* My dreams were less than pleasant.

On day four, again, we didn't see anyone on the trail, and it was another rugged uphill slog. I didn't veer from the trail at all, and never saw any snakes. That night we stopped near a cliff, where we could hear the sounds of water rushing not far away. The guys were comical when preparing the dehydrated dinners, laughing about the difficulty of opening packages, adding water, creating French names for each item, and heating them. We girls gave them a bad time about their name selections, but admitted to each other that this was really a great trip, a great memory making experience for us. After twilight in our campsite, even with the stars in the sky, we could not see our hand out in front of our face without flashlights. I looked forward to nighttime, so snug in my sleeping bag, I could trade fearful thoughts of snakes for restful slumber.

Something woke me from my sleep and I lay there, not moving a muscle. The others slept soundly while I listened. With my heart pounding wildly, I opened my eyes, but couldn't see anything, yet I knew the sound was real and it was getting closer to us. Carefully, I woke John, whispering for him not to move suddenly or make any noises. A few moments later, all of us heard sounds, and understood—bears! They were in our camp, and although we couldn't see them, we could hear our things being torn apart. The bears had a strong dank smell, and we could hear them sniffing, snuffling, snorting, and moving about. Suddenly, a bear moved very close to me. His stench was horrendous as I felt something slimy fall on my arm. I knew it was time to do something; I jumped up and moved away. John yelled in pain, and to scare the bear—the bear had stepped on his leg. In John's haste to get away in the darkness, he stumbled over a log and fell in pain. Although none of us spoke, we knew we were in trouble. I don't know if John's yell frightened the bears, but I was beyond scared, and was having trouble moving because my body was shaking uncontrollably. I've never been as frightened in my life. In the black of night, we four found each other, and cautiously moved away from the camp, hoping we wouldn't fall off the cliff we knew was nearby. We could hear the bears eating but could see nothing. Huddled in the darkness, we experienced a deafening moment of quietness in the numb blackness of our minds, imagining scenarios of what might happen next. We were in mental overload. How many bears were there? How big were they? Would they kill us? We clung together for safety and warmth, and I could feel tears running down Elaine's face. I tried to comfort my injured husband, but I couldn't stop shaking. All of us said silent prayers in the darkness that night. And I prayed for daylight, and for a miracle to get us off the mountain safely. This was the longest, darkest night I had ever spent, and it seemed like an eternity until the dawn began to lighten the sky.

There were no bears around, but our camp was a mess. We soon realized that the guys had not hung our food supply high in the trees, but had put it in our backpacks and leaned them against the trees. The bears had come looking for food, not us. They sucked out whatever was edible, tearing apart anything that could possibly hold a morsel of food. We knew we had a serious problem, since John's leg was broken and he could not walk. Our boots and equipment had been scattered, slobbered on, or torn apart. John was in pain, and we wanted to get him and ourselves off the mountain as fast as possible. More than anything in my life, I did not want to spend another night in the mountain darkness. We had hiked four full days up into the mountains and knew it could take that long to hike out.

Dick made a decision; he would hike to a ranger's station to get help, leaving us girls to care for John. He found both his boots, and then strode off. Elaine and I sat on a log, near John, quiet, motionless, attentive to anything that moved anywhere, and fearing we would have to endure another night of wilderness darkness. John was stretched out on the ground, trying to keep his pain under control by not moving. Our food and water were gone. Fear of darkness and hungry bears dominated my mind, even more than thoughts of snakes. Each of us silently pondered what we had been through, and struggled with our emotions. I wanted to scream . . . *I never wanted to come on this trip!* But, those thoughts just circulated in my mind, not one word escaped to affect John. I was sure each of us wished we had stayed home, or gone to the beach instead of coming on this trip.

As the long hours passed and the daylight faded to darkness, Elaine and I huddled together beside John, and prayed the bears would not come back, and help would arrive soon. We must have slept a little, but by morning, we were hungry and concerned about whether Dick had reached help. About mid morning Dick and a ranger arrived with two horses and an air splint for John. I heaved a huge sigh of relief, until I realized that they were taking John, and not us. I couldn't believe it. The ranger brought us water, nothing else, and told us how to get down by an easy trail, then he and John left by horseback. We three left immediately, and every step of the way, I watched for bears, snakes, or anything else that might come after us. It had taken us four days to hike up—it only took us only one to get down. I moved in record speed, walking, scrabbling, and crawling down large rocks, to get to our car. With each step, I vowed that when I got my boots off, never again would they be on my feet. When safely at the car, I threw my boots in the park trash, along with other things we brought back. I kept only two small, thick Tupperware containers that the bears had sucked food out of as camping mementos.

John's leg had been set by the time we got to the hospital. Now that he was on pain medication and in a warm comfy bed, he greeted us with smiles and jokes about our next trip. I waited until we got home to make it amply clear that I would never go on another back packing trip—not ever. When I put my camping clothes in the trash the following week, I saw him look over at me with the desire to say something, but he had sense enough to not utter a word.

We had been lucky in Tuolumne Meadows, because just a few weeks later, two hikers on the John Muir trail were killed by bears. I thought about our experience and was grateful to be alive. Camping and backpacking is great for those who know and follow the rules of wilderness areas, but for novice campers, and others like me, the adventure can be a disaster. It only took that one backpacking trip to come to a lifelong decision about camping. For me, camping means packing a few casual things, bringing a good book to read and checking into a Holiday Inn, with stars viewable from the balcony of a cozy room with a bed and pillow, while the others enjoy their time in the great outdoors.

Decorating the Christmas Tree

Decorating the Christmas tree has been one of my favorite holiday activities since I was a little girl. I'm not sure if it had to do with anticipating the arrival of Santa Claus or because my mom, dad, and I were doing it together, or maybe because I was trusted to handle the fragile glass ornaments. I looked forward to that night almost as much as Christmas morning.

When I was six years old, we lived in a small Spanish style house in Hawthorne, CA. It was just a block off the main boulevard in town, but the dozen or so homes on our street were clearly residential with small front yards and larger back yards complete with overgrown king palm trees and many lush green lawns with perimeter space for flowerbeds. People in our neighborhood didn't decorate the outside of their homes for Christmas, but they were friendly and sometimes made holiday cookies for one another.

We set aside a specific night to decorate our tree. I vividly remember my mother, just home from work, still wearing her white nurse's uniform, stockings and shoes, climbing a step stool, reaching up into an opening in the ceiling, taking down several old brown boxes, covered with a layer of filthy attic dust. The boxes were filled with Christmas tree decorations that had been bought, collected, or made over the years. While mother changed from her uniform to more comfortable clothes, my dad opened the boxes and pulled out the strings of electric lights. Putting the lights on the tree was the first task, one my parents wouldn't let me help with at that time. I can still see my dad standing on an old metal stool with the look of a man contemplating an important technical job, winding the lights around the top branches of the tree, carefully hiding the wires as much as possible. Mother put the lights on the lower branches of the tree as I stood nearby and watched, eager for them to finish so I could start hanging the pretty ornaments as soon as Dad had the treetop ornament in place. Our tree-topper wasn't too fancy, but it was gold and sparkled more than any other decoration on the tree.

In school, I had made a construction paper chain using all the colors of the rainbow and added to its length at home until it would stretch across the room. While I started unwrapping the ornaments, my dad took one end of the paper chain almost to the top of our tree and wove it around the branches, just as he did the lights. How proud I was of that colorful chain winding from top to bottom.

Because Mother was a "get it done" and "move on" type of personality, she considered the time spent on the tree excessive when she had so many important things to do. Regardless, this was a night Dad and I loved, and refused to rush. My dad's engineering background and desire to get things "right," meant sometimes moving a single glass ornament three or four places to "the perfect spot." That drove Mother crazy, but Dad and

I had lots of fun, laughing and deciding where each would look best. Very few ornaments on our tree were matched; some had dark spots or scratches on them, but hanging together on the tree, they looked stunningly beautiful to me. Once we had hung all the colorful ornaments on the limbs of the tree, we added a few homemade items, then it was time to hang the long silver icicles, one strand at a time. This was more than my mother was willing to do. Glad to be finished with her part of the project, she went to the kitchen to prepare hot chocolate for us, and cookies, if there were any. While waiting for us, she stood in the kitchen near the doorway where she could listen to our chatter and watch, while polishing then buffing her white nurse's shoes. She was meticulous about her appearance, always leaving for work looking like she just stepped out of a magazine. When she had finished her shoes and was ready for another days work, she settled in a chair, read the Christmas cards, and then began hanging them, one by one with straight pins, on the stationary panels of our large floral printed living room draperies.

When done dressing the tree, we gathered in the living room with our cups of hot chocolate, turned the house lights off, then on cue, turned on the tree lights to admire our work. It was a magical moment, and though it was late when we finished, and bedtime for me, I went to sleep thinking about our beautiful Christmas tree.

Both my parents were well educated, had good jobs, and were saving money to buy a house, so they didn't spend much for holiday decorations while living in Hawthorne. When I was eight, we moved to a newly constructed house in Downey, CA. It was in a new housing development and most of the neighbors were involved with planting trees and putting in grass to eliminating the dirt that came indoors with the wind, or from happy but dirty feet. At our house, the first thing Mother chose then ordered were the living room draperies, which were a smooth, luxurious looking white fabric with a pleated valance of the same fabric. As the Christmas cards arrived that year and many years following, Mother following tradition, carefully pinned each card to the bottom edge of the valance.

As I got older, my dad and I became more and more particular about choosing the Christmas tree itself, and would go from lot to lot checking out every tree, trying to find "the perfect one." Mother chose to stay home and get the decorations out while we went on our quest. Not only did we come home with trees that stood from floor to ceiling, we came home with stories of our search that only *we* could appreciate. Because of the time we spent choosing the tree and bringing it home, our tree decorating labor of love, now took over two days, with one day to get the tree, and the other to decorate it. Even so, always, at the end of our decorating, we gathered as a family with our hot chocolate, then the house lights were turned off and the Christmas tree lights switched on, for us all to admire and enjoy our creation.

Our holiday traditions continued and expanded. After the first Christmas, this new neighborhood put decorations outside, too, and most neighbors ran

Christmas lights on the eaves of their roofing, so we followed suit. Then one year my mother found a Mr. and Mrs. Snowman pattern. My dad cut them out of sheets of plywood, and we all helped paint them. They stood like a family in our front yard during the month of December and got quite a lot of attention in the neighborhood. We were so proud of them. The homes on a street close to us stacked three large spray painted rounds of tumbleweed on top of each other, and put snowman hats and scarves on them. The entire street was decorated as if by a cookie cutter—all the same. Night after night, cars drove slowly around the neighborhood to see what our neighborhood had done to celebrate the Christmas season.

Those childhood years have long passed, but the memories and joy of decorating the Christmas tree continues. My husband has little interest in spending hours decorating the tree but goes with me to pick it out and helps set it up. Sometimes we put our tree in the 20 foot high entry of our house, and other times we put it upstairs in our bedroom in front of the picture windows facing the main channel, where other homes and tour boats can see the lights twinkle from afar. He helps me string the lights on the top branches, then excuses himself, so I can begin decorating, spending hours getting ornaments and the treasures made by our children and grandchildren placed just right. Over the years, I have gathered beautiful elegant ornaments and ribbons for a more formal look on our tree, and have boxes of old sentimental ornaments we used when the children were little, or that we gathered while traveling. Once I have decided on the type of ornaments to use, those boxes of ornaments are brought down from our storeroom. I then start a favorite holiday movie on DVD, and enjoy decorating the tree. As daylight dims and darkness sets in, I turn on the twinkle lights already wound through the tree branches for a couple of seconds before turning the regular house lights on. Then I just sit and look at them, twinkling and blinking like the stars in the sky.

I love the fragrance of freshly cut Scotch pine or noble fir from our tree permeating throughout our home, more so when the needles begin drying out and the fragrance intensifies. Each year, it is with a twinge of remorse that I un-decorate the tree, put the ornaments back in their containers for another year, and drag the Christmas tree out to the trash area for pick up.

Only three years in my life have I skipped this beautiful night of decorating, each while I cared for my parents who knew not the season and my heart was involved in attending to them. Now that they have passed away, I again look forward to decorating, as much or more, never forgetting those special memories of years past when we were so young and did it together. Those were *good ole days,* replaced by many other memorable times, such as when I put finishing touches on our Christmas tree, with my grandchildren helping on the lower branches, or assembling the tracks for the electric train to run around it. How I love the sounds of their happy voices talking with each other, about what section they will complete, then the fun watching the train go round and round, sometimes just missing a low hanging branch, or an ornament on the tree.

One December, when we were expecting our grand-children to come stay for the weekend, we put a smaller second tree upstairs in our bedroom so they could set up the train around the tree then sleep on the floor near it. I was always grateful to have the children with us, and wanting this time to be especially memorable, we all bunched up in our pajamas on top of our bed, and threw artificial snow and pieces of torn quilt-batting onto the tree, pretending it was snowing in the forest. We had so much fun that night and together decided, for that year, it was enough, so not a single decoration went on the tree. That night we had hot chocolate, watched a Christmas cartoon movie, and talked about our special tree, without lights or bulbs.

The joys of decorating the Christmas tree continue in my life. When that task gets to be too much for me, I'll pray to be taken back to my Father in Heaven, and I will look over anyone who needs a guardian angel to help them find joy, decorating their Christmas tree.

"Mother, Where Are You?"

When I look back on the past ten years of my life and think of all the exciting things I have done, the many places I have been, the never ending family times I treasure, I wonder why one circumstance surfaces over all the others.

After a lifetime of caring for others and staying active, my mother's personality made dramatic changes. She started repeating herself, got lost in her favorite stories, and became paranoid, hostile, and violent. We were at our wits end, and I made an appointment with a dementia and Alzheimer's counselor at the John Douglas French Center in Los Alamitos for my mother, father, husband Jerry, and myself. The counselor had seen both my parents several times, so that day we were all there to talk with him together and separately. During my private moments with the counselor, he told me frankly that putting my mother in an Alzheimer's care center could escalate my father's demise from grief as quickly as if I let them remain at home and have her batter him to death.

While I sat with my mother waiting for her turn, the counselor hurried out of his office to call an ambulance because my dad was having chest pains and complained his heart was beating erratically. The hospital was called. Then mother's psychiatrist (from her former hospitalization) and the counselor arranged with the staff to have my dad taken to emergency to be cared for, then under the pretense of taking mother to see my dad, attendants would come get mother and lead her into locked door hospitalization. Jerry drove my mother and me to the hospital, and it seemed like it took forever to get there. Mother was unable to stay focused on anything, making our time with her difficult. Arriving at the hospital, we were told that Dad was being examined in Critical Care, and almost immediately, the psych-unit was there to get mother. We had tried for months to get her to a doctor for her anger, memory, and personality issues. Our problem was that she knew enough as a nurse in her earlier days of decline to know what evaluation meant for her, and had refused all help. Now, finally, she was going behind locked doors for evaluation, and long overdue placement.

Jerry and I sat alone in the emergency room lobby that night for almost an hour, in a state of numbness and disbelief at what had just transpired—thinking, it couldn't be happening—but it just had. For days afterwards, we each mulled over what had taken place that day, that night, and the years prior. The event we all knew would happen *some day,* had happened. It was past tense now, with Mother under doctor's care, where we hoped she would be medicated and *calm enough for us to just be with her,* without the violence her illness had triggered.

Nevertheless, guilty thoughts lingered. Was it the right move? Did I do the right thing? It sure didn't feel right. I'm not sure that in my lifetime I will ever completely recover from that night and having to make that decision. I hope I do, but it still haunts me.

The Care Center called me because Mother needed clothes from underwear to pajamas. I drove to her house, looked in her drawers, then in her closet. Sorting through her clothing was such an eerie experience for me, because I felt like I was doing something I shouldn't. Mother had been so meticulous about her clothes, and I admired her for that trait. As I pushed each hanger to the side, I was truly shocked at how the depth of her illness was so visible in her closet.

All my life, my mother told me stories of her childhood and the poverty she grew up in. She hated it, and had a hard time seeing the blessings and love woven in her large family. All she remembered was that her clothes were made from itchy feed sacks, and how she resented being teased about having the sack label show somewhere. She also recalled the hand-me-down clothes given to her family, which her mother remade into school clothes for her and her four sisters. Many times the material was of a fabric like satin, inappropriate for school clothes, but in those poor times, any material at all was better than none. Such memories festered in Mother's heart and mind, as did the resentments that some of her sisters weren't careful with their communal clothes, and would rip their dresses or get stains on them, even knowing they would have to take turns wearing them—soiled or not. Mother hated that. Then a trip to her aunt's home in Cincinnati, Ohio, changed her life forever. Her aunt had a large home with electric lights, a maid, a car, and beautiful clothing. That trip made her more determined than ever to work hard, have stylish clothing, and have all the nice things that money would buy. She was never happy at home again. She worked many jobs to earn money, and left for nursing school as soon as she could.

Mother proudly worked as a registered nurse all her life, and she took great pride in her spotless white uniforms. On her days off, she always put on clean clothing and she loved fine cotton fabrics. Mother's past structured for her life, and her need to have immaculate tailored clothing, polished shoes, and well coiffed hair. As long as she lived, she vowed she would never be caught dead looking as poorly dressed as she remembered her mother looking long ago.

So as I moved from one dress to another, tears trickled down my cheeks as I saw her clothing. Dress after dress was a reminder of just how sick she had become just from the way she had hung her clothes, mismatched and dirty, with jackets, blouses, skirts, and dresses askew. Some were inside out, others on top of each other, belts of one print with dresses of another style. It was like opening a wound to see how far she had degenerated into this horrible all encompassing Alzheimer's disease, realizing how it had affected her judgment. Many of her clothes were stained and her shoes told the same story, scuffed and badly in need of cleaning and polish. Everything in her closet just screamed out, something is wrong! My mother, the proud nurse and one of the cleanest women I ever knew, was gone, and the goals which she worked and lived for, no longer existed.

I piled many of her things in the trunk of my car as quickly as I could, so I wouldn't upset my dad, who himself had just come home from the hospital and was trying to cope with his loss, his disappointment in not being able to help her, and his relief to be able to sleep and sit in peace without worrying about mother coming to harm him. Half of his life was gone after over 50 years together. He mourned for his loss and hated himself for not having more patience with Mother, for not being able to protect her, for breaking his promise to never put her in a home, and for losing control and saying mean things to strike back during her vicious attacks. He was wounded too, mentally, and physically. I closed my car trunk and carried on a generic conversation with my dad for an hour or so as if Mother was just out somewhere. Neither of us could talk about her without tears streaming down our faces and our hearts breaking. We kept up good fronts for each other, and I left, mid-afternoon, for home.

As I drove home, a deep sadness overcame me and tears flowed as if a dam had been opened. I felt like a fool, hoping people in the cars besides me wouldn't think a psycho was next to them as I sobbed and sobbed. That day I prayed for God to just get me home.

Though I knew my mother was now hospitalized where she would get constant care, I felt such a loss, a guilt for not being able to help her; then relief that the inevitable decision had been made and executed. I didn't know what the future held for any of us, especially Mother, but I did know she was where people could watch her, and care for her without the emotional attachment and the physical abuse that my dad and I took for many agonizing years, as we watched her deteriorate and vocalize her hate towards us.

I called several times each day to check with the nurses to see how mother was doing. She was a handful; almost daily, something triggered a violent, angry, day when they had to lock her up for several hours. Sometimes I could hear her screaming from lockdown, and it broke my heart. I wanted to rush right down there and rescue my mother from this hell. They would let her out of isolation if she would take her medication, but she would only do it with much prodding and anger. Then magically, a few hours later she was in the dining room eating with the others. She needed medication so badly but was so resistant to taking any. My head knows that no matter what we did to try to make Mother happy, had she been home those same violent days would have taken place with my dad and me being attacked. Logically, I knew it was the disease taking over, but my heart broke that I couldn't be with my mother and help her as she had always done for me. It broke my heart that she was alive, breathing, locked up and my presence caused her extreme distress. I never knew if I would ever get to visit her again and have her be happy I had come to see her. I don't know if she will ever know how much I tried to help her, show my love and admiration for her. I hope someday I will know, she knows I love her, and . . . I will know. . . . She loved me!

I have relived that incident many times since 1998, and still feel sadness over her loss of freedom and life. She rarely recognized me. Sometimes she told me about her daughter and a couple of times said to me "I like you," and I wanted to jump with joy. She died in 2002, a fragile 86-pound woman that I scarcely recognized but would love forever.

Paul "Sammy" Larkin

I have a theory about writers: some are born storytellers, and others must learn how to tell stories. I have a theory about stories: they give us knowledge that is unobtainable through other media or genres. In what seems decades ago, Linda Flower did a study of how experts (for instance, lawyers) "decipher" difficult texts. She found that they narratize, turning the exposition into stories. As I recall, one of the difficult texts was regulations for marine radios, and the reader of this text did something like this: "Let's see, if I have a boat and want to apply for a radio license, then I have to. . . ." Robert de Beaugrande convincingly demonstrated that data embedded in a narrative is more readily understood and remembered longer than data presented in tabular form or in exposition. In other words, there is something powerful and powerfully human about stories. (The Bible is powerful, not because of its theology, but because it is a collection of stories.)

A storyteller has a visual imagination, supplying readers with the tremendous trifles that add up to verisimilitude and a kind of wisdom. Paul Larkin is a storyteller.

—W.R.W.

"Ole George" and the Paper Boy

Sixty some years ago, I lived in Amory, Mississippi, a town of about 4,000 that had sprouted along the Frisco Railroad line, halfway between Memphis, Tennessee, and Birmingham, Alabama. It was in Amory, and I was fifteen, when I decided to enter a Seminary.

Knowing that to send me to the Seminary at this early age might be somewhat costly for my parents, I looked around for summer jobs to help pay some of the costs. I inquired of the Commercial Appeal newspaper—the big one out of Memphis, TN—as to whether they might need a boy to cover a paper route in our neighborhood. They did have an opening, for two months of the summer vacation, and it was for the north section of Amory, the very area in which we lived. Super! This job would cover only two very early hours of each day, thus leaving me time to do other work for income. I tossed newspapers in early mornings, often dark, through rain, sleet, cold, heat, and even a few fine days.

At four-thirty every morning, I'm jumping on my trusty bike, and peddling two miles to the railroad station to pick up my bundles of papers. My route covered the northerly section of Amory, including several homes on a highway that stretches a ways beyond our fine community. Besides the usual dogs chasing me along the way, slick icy surfaces, and occasional nasty wind blown rain soaking me, my job was like that experienced by thousands of stalwart paper delivery boys and girls throughout our country.

Following is a short story of my experience delivering the bulky, early Sunday edition of the paper throughout the entire town, together with a black man and his mule, Ole George.

Delivering the Sunday edition of the Commercial Appeal provided me a somewhat unique experience. What was special about Sunday deliveries was *Ole George.* He was a medium size brown mule of indeterminate age, who with head bowed to the yoke was hardly distinguishable from any other old mule, but for one special distinction; Ole George knew the paper route, the entire route, throughout the town. His owner was a small unassuming black man of few words and quiet manner, from the *Sticks*—that is from across the tracks where all the Negro folk lived as opposed to our side of the tracks where all the white residents lived. Well, we three would pick up our huge stack of papers, pile them on the mule's low flat wagon with rubber tires to keep noise down, and head out.

Will—all mature black men were called Will in the South at that time—would call out, "Gee" to Ole George, and that mute mule would start his steady mosey down the middle of the street. What was a wonder for me, was that Ole George pulled the cart such that Will and I, at the rear of the wagon, could fold and toss out papers to each side of the street, and without being given any signal, continue going straight, or turn right or left. And yep, Ole George would even slow down or speed up to keep pace with us while we put papers onto the porches of our sleeping customers. I was truly in awe of that *dern smart-alick ole mule,* for outside of my delivery area, I had no idea of the route throughout the entire town. But that mule, Ole George, sure did. and with each early Sunday morning lesson from him, I learned, better than from any church sermon, the lesson of humility, and a smidgeon of admiration and respect for those beasts of burden, my brothers, the mule.

Amory Library

I am an unabashed Book Nut. What a grand passion.

Books have fascinated me from my earliest childhood, at two to three years old. Those flat little bright books—picture books, coloring books, those teaching ABC's and numbers, describing animals, and the world beyond my view—made me realize I was coming into endless discovery. We had stacks of those precious little intriguing sources of information, and I treasured them. I was about four when I found several boxes of dusty old hardbound grownup books in our garage. One with black and white pictures was a Bible history book. The pictures were of a very unappealing landscape with barren stone structures. For the life of me, I couldn't understand why anyone could or would live in such a desolate environment with no trees or plants of any kind. I did my best to decipher the print found under each picture, but, puzzle as I might, it was to no avail.

It was frustrating not to be able to find the key to reading. I took one book to Mom for perhaps some enlightenment. "Now Sammy, go away and find all those colored books in the closet. Don't bother me with this. I don't have time for it right now." It was then I realized I needed to go to school like my older sister, Mary Ann, and learn to read. Therefore, I began pestering my parents to allow me to go to school.

At five, I was in the first grade, and learning how to read. Alleluia! At seven I entered the third grade and received a further impetus toward books. The teaching nun treated me so badly that year that I learned to hate school—with a terrible passion—yet my desire to learn was undiminished. This traumatic experience compelled me almost exclusively toward books as the source of my learning instruction.

From the third grade on through graduation from high school, and beyond, books were my constant companions. I read one class's literature book from cover to cover, and then jump to the next class's literature book. I could never get enough reading.

In the summer of 1944 when I was 12 years old, someone told me that our small town of Amory, Mississippi had a lending library upstairs in a two story commercial building on Main Street. This I had to explore. I jumped on my bike and peddled the one-mile to Main Street. Sure enough, I found a tiny sign, LIBRARY, next to narrow steep wooden stairs leading to the second story. The door was open and in I went with the excitement of a kid slipping under a Christmas tree early in the morning. For me this was a dreamland, rows of bookshelves full from top to bottom with my friends, just begging me to pick them up and get to know what they were all about. I could hardly contain myself as I entered that door. I don't think I had ever been in a real library before and was somewhat overwhelmed, bewildered with the awesome possibilities before me. Where to start?

Man! I just started by pulling out the first book I came to on the shelf next to the door. Well, I found in a hurry that this wouldn't do. There were three ladies looking at me, the older fat one sitting at a tiny desk stopped me dead, asking me, "What are you looking for? Boy!" At first, I was at a loss to answer, for it seemed obvious to me, I was here to look at books, hundreds and hundreds of precious volumes. I just wanted to lose myself, right here and now, and stay till closing time, and then be back first thing next morning to immerse myself again till I had consumed every book in this place. Oh, no! Right off, I found that's not how these ladies operated.

"You put that book back, carefully, right in the same place you got it. Now come over here to my desk, and let me talk to you. What's your name? BOY!" She didn't say boy very sweetly though, so I knew she meant business.

I was perplexed, thinking, why did this lady with her mean-haughty look have to be so bossy? Can't she be nice? I know these books are not mine, and are precious and are public property. I wouldn't harm one page in this entire room. You see, I LOVE books and treasure them, every one of them whether I would read them or not.

She got my name, address, and phone number, my parent's name, how old I was and what grade I was in.

I think she would have given me a body search right there if she'd thought of it. The other two heavy ladies hovering over her shoulder were glaring at me. I truly felt a bit intimidated and began to feel guilty, but for the life of me I didn't know why. Maybe they thought I was there to case the joint and would come back later and burn the place down. Did they think that their whole purpose in life there was to protect *their* property from my destructive intent?

"You have to get a Library Card."

"Why? I just came in to see what you have up here."

"What're you looking for then?"

"Gosh, I don't know until I look around." Hadn't these ladies ever just gone shopping until they finally found something of interest?

"Children's books are over there."

"Why must I limit myself to juvenile books? Ain't I twelve years old?" Well, did I get a couple of smirks and whispered comments from behind the back of their hands, together with definitive shakes of the head.

"Listen, young man, if you're going to talk to us like that you can just turn around and walk out that door."

"No Ma'am, I mean no disrespect. I just heard about your being up here with all these books and thought I might take a look-see. I mean no harm."

"Well then, you can go over to that shelf and look, but be careful and don't turn down the corner of any pages."

What the hell does she take me for, anyway? I was so nervous and overwrought at this point that the first book I pulled out of the shelf I almost dropped. It was a good thing I played baseball, catching it before it hit the floor, and they didn't see me do it. I'll bet that if I hadn't rescued that valuable Edgar Rice Burrows book *Son of Tarzan,* those ladies would have called the police on me and I would have been thrown in jail.

At that point, I thought, maybe I better not stay around here much longer where I'm obviously not welcome. I really just wanted to explore, delve into this wondrous jungle, and discover the riches I knew without doubt were hidden within. Oh well, I started for the door, to escape, with the book in hand. But, no!

"Where are you going with that book?"

"I was just talking it home to read. I'll bring it back, really."

"Don't you know you need to sign out with a library card before you can take a book from the library?"

"No Ma'am. This is my first time. I've never ever done this before."

It cost me 50 cents to sign up, a lot of money for me at that time. I rarely had that much money in my pocket either. Luckily, I had just come from mowing a neighbor's yard and had come straight here to check out this place. Maybe my being dirty and smelly is why these blue-nosed ladies are so high and mighty, and treating me so mean.

"We have rules here you know," the first lady was saying. "Now you keep that book clean, don't get it wet and return in within one week. I'll stamp in with the return date and if you bring it back late, you will pay a fine."

She went on and on, till my head was spinning with all their regulations. Didn't she have my hard earned 50 cents? Why—that was about the value of the book.

I was dizzy and a bit sick and my belly felt funny as I road my bike home. I had ridden this route for years and could do anything on these wheels, but I sure was shaky going home that day.

I really enjoyed that Tarzan book, and from my lawn mowing work, I even purchased a companion volume, *Tarzan of the Apes*. Well, I was late returning that book, so we got notices and threats in the mail, but I was never going back to that place to be humiliated and treated so. With my brothers, I went off to boarding school in Arkansas in September. I guess Mom took that book back, I don't know for sure, nor did I really care. Those ladies with their attitude had more rules than Carter had liver pills. The town's library was hardly larger than a normal sized bedroom, yet those old biddies made like it was their *Taj Mahal*.

When I got back the next summer from boarding school, those two Tarzan books had disappeared down some dark hole. This became a yearly pattern with my books. Therefore, I resolved that when I grew up, I would build my own library and, no one had better mess with MY BOOKS!

One more memory about books. One evening in the early 1940s, Dad came home with what was for us children, *a gift from the gods,* a beat up old gray-backed set of the Encyclopedia Britannica. I loved those books, going through them over and over, especially in the winter and when the weather was bad outside. I could never get enough of those books, the pleasure they gave seemed inexhaustible. If I had not a love for books and reading before they were brought into the home, then they certainly cemented that love.

My opinion is often stated as: "A Home Without Books is a House Without a Soul."

"Tick"

This brief true story treats a subject that is a bit delicate for me to attempt to properly relate. Well—see, it's a mite personal. Matter of fact it could hardly get more personal—to the point—it has to do with the very *tip* of a certain protuberance which boys keep hidden (for the most part) from the rest of the world. Well, let me take a deep breath and take the plunge.

You see, I loved to tramp in the Mississippi woods and the wide-open spaces, and that being so, I did expose myself to all kinds of critters which might attack me. Such as the usual: mosquitoes, rats, snakes, bees of all kinds, leeches, stinging ants; and stinging nettles, poison ivy, and—well, you get the message—and I even acquired a parasite.

But, where exactly did I pick up this dastardly parasite? I'm not sure. I believe I had gone fishing and while waiting for a bite had got bitten. Not on my arms, not on my legs but . . . Gosh, how to say it?

I first noticed it when I was walking home from the lake (fishless, but had unknowingly caught something) and began to feel a funny little itch, and in an increasingly insistent manner. The more I walked the more irritating it became, till by the time I got home there was an almost fiery stinging—very uncomfortable. In the bathroom, I couldn't wait to pull my pants down to find out what the source of this exceeding discomfiture was.

I was about 12 or 13 at the time, and at that age a boy can be very sensitive and self-conscious about matters of this nature. First, I thought it was just a twig that had fallen down my shirt, somehow worked its way into my shorts, and was irritating me around my crotch. Now I had to empty my bladder and I almost choked when I found the true source of my problem— it was much worse than I could have imagined.

There, embedded inside the very tip of the most tender and delicate orifice of my young body, hanging, clamped, head and claws buried halfway in my pink defenseless aperture—was a disgusting, potentially dangerous and infectious invading TICK.

I was terrified. I didn't want to call Mother, but what was I to do? "Mom! I need Daddy—and *right now!*"

"What's the matter, Sammy?"

"Mom! Just call Daddy and have him come from work right now. It's very important," I said, piteously through the locked bathroom door, and choking tears as I held my tortured member in a panicked embrace.

"Sammy, tell me what in the world is bothering you so I can tell your Dad."

"Just get him, Mom. I've been bitten by something."

"Unlock this door and let me see."

"No!"

I don't know if I had ever seen this type of insect before, but I was becoming too knowledgeable about it with its exceedingly intimate proximity. Each time I looked at that loathsome thing clinging to the end of my *——the intrusive loathsome predator seemed to be getting bigger, and it wasn't just my imagination. As I watched and waited for Dad to come home the two miles from work to help me, that damn thing's body was actually swelling up before my eyes, like a miniature gray balloon filling itself with my rich red blood. Now I was learning what bloated really meant, first hand.

God, I was scared. When Dad got home and surveyed my predicament, he could hardly suppress his enormous amusement, despite my obvious overwhelming discomfiture.

His *remedy*—was a regular darning needle from Mom's sewing basket, he heated the tip of the needle till it was red hot with the flame of a match. With serious mien and at the same time trembling with suppressed amusement, Dad went about the delicate business of attempting to extract the tick's buried head from my bodily extension in such a manner as to prevent the head breaking off inside my skin and so preclude infection. At that point I was probably screaming, thinking I would be burnt and deformed—ruined for life, he carefully laid the red-hot needle on the back of this glutted bloodsucker.

The thing moved, and Dad gently pulled it from my skin, and crushed it, blood squirting between his fingers and then flushed the disgusting deflated remains down the toilet, and washed his hands.

What an ordeal. I was sobbing with fear, frustrated, embarrassed, and wondering what eternal damage had been inflicted to the end of my red swollen member, and wincing as it was being dabbed, gingerly but searingly, with an alcohol soaked cloth to disinfect this now-burning area.

The point of attack became a flaming blood blister (later a dark maroon color) that gradually, over literally years, diminished in size and eventually disappeared. I wondered often, while a green teenager, had that red mark persisted, whether it might affect, or in some way hinder, other *activities* of my growing manhood.

Let me hold the answer to that question for some other essay.

Baseball Long Toss Contest

At the end of my first full year in Amory High School, I was surprised by a year-end tradition that had been established there, a field competition by the entire student body. The activities were of many kinds for girls and boys—running, jumping, football throwing, tumbling, baton twirling—and about any kind of physical challenge they could dream up. Coming on to this unexpectedly, I was not prepared to enter into the fun until the baseball throwing trial came up.

My brothers Jimmy, Johnny, and I had many times crossed our street to the empty elementary school playground to toss a baseball, using the new beautiful leather ball gloves that our parents had given to us for our birthdays. Besides catching for Johnny, who was practicing as a pitcher, we also exercised our throwing arms, testing to see how far we could toss that little ball from one end of that long field to the other, endlessly. We thought we were pretty good, but we had no way of knowing how we compared with others our age.

After watching the ball throwing trials awhile, I figured I might not do too bad and so stepped forward and got in line. It seemed almost every boy in the school wanted to get into this single elimination competition, throwing that ball as far as they could from one end of the football field to the other, 300 feet or more. It soon became obvious that the test was coming down to only two contestants; Tommy Longnecker, the six-foot two inch and about 200 pound captain of our football team, senior class president, and the all round most handsome and popular student in the school, against the practically unknown and ignored first-year junior student and *Yankee,* Sammy Larkin.

Tommy was the youngest son of the well-known Longnecker family, who owned and operated the large and most successful garment factory located on the south edge of town, where they hired more employees than any other business enterprise in our small town of about 4,000 population.

Tommy had thrown early and had established the mark to beat, which no one had yet come near. Being at the end of the line I finally stepped forward as a few observers began to move off for the next competition of the day. I wondered if all that practice with my brothers was going to pay off or not. With a couple of warm up tosses, I finally was ready for my throw. With two long jump steps forward, I let go of that ball down the field with all my might. I thought the three referees at the other end of the field were taking an inordinate amount of time judging my ball, but finally their sign went up informing us that my last ball thrown had rolled a few feet beyond Tommy's mark. That news created an instant electric stir about us, and caused the judges to go into *conference*. The outcome of their decision was that Tommy and I should have a three-ball-each play-off to determine the winner of this competition. The first balls we each had already tossed would stand as our first throw.

At once, there was evinced a great deal of interest in this competition with a crowd gathering about us. Tommy was chosen to make his second toss. When Tommy had stepped up for his initial toss, it was with casualness, even perhaps with a certain bravado. Now, readying himself for his second toss, though a bit more serious, he yet showed his usual confident assurance in his superior ability. With a couple of quick skips forward, he launched his ball in a high long arc down the field. Almost immediately loud whoops came from the other end of the field and the referees sign popped up with the new measurement showing that Tommy's ball had out distanced Sammy's by a yard or so. The crowd around us cheered with excitement as their hero, smil-

PAUL "SAMMY" LARKIN

ing broadly, stepped aside to be lost amid his adoring admirers.

As I readied myself for my second toss, I realized that I had to adjust my throw so that my ball must arc a bit higher to get more distance toward that far goal post. Winding up I let go of the ball with all my might, it rising up as I had planned, and reaching out to that beckoning distance. The three judges at the other end scurried about a bit longer this time, before recording their numbers on their clipboard, and finally, their big sign went up showing that Sammy's ball had outdistanced Tommy's by hardly a foot or two. No cheer went up; rather a low moan greeted the announcement of the results, yet it bothered me not at all for had this not ever been the case with me and our family here in Amory? There was now a real challenge for the crowd's champion, and with only one ball each yet to be sent skyward from the contestants, we all could feel the tension; it was palpable.

The third and last ball was now handed to Tommy, and as he looked at it for a long second he knew that this was it, for he must win or forever face embarrassment and humiliation for losing to Larkin. This was serious! Standing tall then, this superb athletic young man straightened his back, readying himself for this defining moment, as his eyes and mind calculated the demand he must make on himself to win this challenge. As the taut, fluid muscular movements of a superbly conditioned body must, Tommy's legs arms and torso leapt forward at his brain's command to heave that leather bound ball far into the deep azure blue sky.

76

Young boys broke from the assembled watchers racing along the side of the football field following that ball to its final place of rest. It was excitement uncontained. Clearly, his ball had gone beyond all others, there was no doubt. There was no containing the joy of the on-lookers, but wait, there was one last ball yet to be sent aloft—Sammy's.

When the excitement had somewhat settled, Sammy, taking the final ball from an official, stepped up to the mark. The crowd was now quiescent with the exception of an occasional muffled taunt. For the first time, I felt a bit nervous, with a tightening in my stomach, and dryness in my throat. How could I best this Adonis, Tommy? I had to calm myself, yet not lose the needed tension of the adrenalin rush. With all the cool reserve I could summon up, I steeled myself to throw the ball a mile, and I would do it. My whole body, with all its energy flowing powerfully toward the mark, as with rocket force Sammy released that ball on its fateful course. It sailed higher and farther than I thought I might ever have been able to send it. And now I could but wait the outcome of my mighty effort, and the three judges' measurements and report.

The judges were far distant down that field, and took an unusual amount of time with what looked like their taking a second look and measurement, and a consultation meeting. The crowd was beginning to become restless on our end of the field. Finally, we saw the fateful sign go up. TOMMY, it read. With that, a huge screaming cheer went up like you wouldn't be-lieve. There was joy and laughing and pounding on backs. Their Adonis, their Samson, their Hero had prevailed: *The South had Risen again.*

Tommy, standing next to me, turned with his hand held out saying, with uncommon seriousness as he looked into my eyes and shook my hand, "Thank you." No one else spoke with me as I shuffled slowly through those milling students the two lonely blocks home that afternoon as confusing and questioning thoughts filled my heated brain. I couldn't help reflecting and wondering to myself why were not the final measurements recorded on the Judges' clipboard and posted clearly on their sign and held high for all to see? And why was there such obvious confusion down under the goal posts there at the end, and why did it take them so much time to report their findings? A parting shot, on what was the last day I would ever see either the teachers or students of Amory High School.

Knockout Punch

A little intro to this story seems appropriate. My parents were strong Catholics who had made tremendous sacrifices to see that their three daughters and three sons received a sound Catholic education. Since we lived in Amory, a small Mississippi town that was practically all Protestant, in the rural South. we were all sent out of state for our Catholic schooling. Father and mother did something special for my senior year of high school, and sent my two brothers and me to St. Agnes Catholic High School where they had graduated in their hometown of Springfield, Missouri. The entire family participated in preparing for this event and we were sent off with high ideals and expectations.

At St. Agnes Catholic High School, each school day began with religious services, Mass and Communion, and a Homily and Prayer. So it was with complete shock and disbelief when the day after we boys stocked our gym lockers with our hard earned and expensive exercise clothes, that we found we had been robbed—our lockers emptied. All of our gym clothes, underwear, shirts, shorts, socks and shoes—everything—gone.

I was so shocked, horrified, and in disbelief, that I rebelled, telling those in charge I would have nothing to do with acquiring replacements for the stolen items, nor would I, in any way, participate in any of the school's gym activities. Thereafter, I sat high in the bleachers in the gym, reading a book, ignoring all the activities on the floor below, wanting nothing more than to be left alone during this class hour. This may help to explain what precipitated the following confrontation.

Our Parish Priest, short, rugged, balding, cigar chomping Father V. A. Schroeger, who I liked in a respectful *father figure* way, and the school's tall mature basketball coach, Robert Taylor, were on the court below talking with some of the boys. A sharp gruff, imperious, "Sammy, get down here," from Father Schroeger broke into my reading concentration. Complying quickly to join the gathering, I guessed immediately the implication of the two pairs of dark brown boxing gloves that both the Father and the coach had in their hands. Without introduction or preliminaries, the coach grabbed my arm and proceeded to force my hand into a glove. I must have stepped back in my surprise, asking, "What's this all about? I don't want to fight anyone."

"Oh, but you do," responded the coach, "and you will."

"Wait," I said, "I don't want to hurt anyone." With that, a loud derisive laugh rose from the gathering crowd of boys about us. It was quite a joke I guess, for the other pair of gloves was being slipped on and tied to John Swift's hands. Why pick as my opponent, a quiet, likeable young man who came from a well known local farm family, and was just about the huskiest boy in our senior class, a natural football lineman.

Till then I had never had a fight unless it were to protect myself or one of my brothers, and then only when I was forced to it. Nobody here except my two brothers knew that our father, a well trained boxer himself, had trained us, and well, that we might defend ourselves from those aggressive *Rebel* boys in the South who constantly had been hassling us since our move to Mississippi from Missouri. I had never had a fight just for sport and didn't like the idea at all. Here I was with no choice but to fight, whether I wanted it or not. Why are they doing this to me? I wondered. It was bewildering.

I didn't like the whole scene, it just didn't seem right. I was clad in my regular school clothes, with only socks on my feet. The gym floor was hard and slick, and there was no defined and controlled area in which to box; besides, they gave us no parameters. Just looking at the way John held his arms, told me he knew little about boxing. I decided, that being quick, I could just spar around John for awhile, keeping him at a safe distance by throwing light punches at him, keeping this up until they hopefully called a halt to this ridiculous farce. I had no intention of really hitting him hard on any portion of his ample body, or hurting him in any way. There was no reason to.

Our maneuvering around went on for a couple of minutes, with my plan working smoothly until, getting careless, I allowed John to connect a powerful long *round house* punch to the side of my head—BLAM! I received a surprisingly heavy blow, momentarily stunning me; I literally did see stars. Dancing away from his long heavy arms to regain my balance and clear my head, I realized he was still coming at me, now with even more force and energy. He had really slipped one to me. I had to call a stop to this quickly! I couldn't take a *score* like that again.

I now attacked John furiously in a way I had not previously done, throwing a flurry of fast left punches to his surprised face. With this he stepped back startled, dropping his guard, giving me the exact opening I was seeking. Suddenly, WHUMP! I connected, with all my might, one-straight-solid-right to the point of his jaw and that was all it took. John, instantly an inert mass, like a big sack of potatoes, went down—THUD! He hit the hardwood floor, down for the count—out cold—end of fight.

An amazed gasp arose from those crowded around, he fell so fast I know they must have thought I had killed him. The coach and Father Schroeger were down on the floor trying to bring him around, and it did take them some time with a wet towel to his face, before he finally sat up, dazed. Once they unlaced and had the gloves off both of us, they must have tossed them into the incinerator for they were never seen again. Boxing was never again on the list of sports at that school, nor did anyone there ever again seem to wish to challenge me to a bout or even mention the incident in my presence. So much for Sammy's first and last *fight event* at St. Agnes High School. In retrospect, I think thereafter there must have been, stemming from this incident, understandably from some, a certain residue of resentment toward me, an outsider that year. I didn't give up my reading, however!

The Ring

Following our football season, in which the three Larkin brothers participated intensely, the school now turned to basketball. Both Johnny and Jimmy had played basketball in boy's boarding school in Arkansas for several years and were pretty good at it, so they joined the teams. I had not participated in this activity with them, so I decided to try boxing, a sport I thought I might do well in and enjoy. For, had not our father boxed, and had not one of his brothers, Uncle Jimmy, become an outstanding Featherweight professional at one time, down in Louisiana in the 1920s?

After an unfortunate knockout I had delivered to one of my fellow students in our school gym early in my senior year at St. Agnes, I received a call from a representative of the town's '449' Boxing Club, asking if I might be interested in coming down for an interview to possibly join their group as a Golden Gloves boxer. So one afternoon I made my way down to the huge Shrine Mosque Auditorium at the edge of the City's business district, then to the basement where the club's work out facility was located. After a short meeting with the club manager, he took me through their large gym, where young men and boys were exercising vigorously in the ring, as well as using a range of boxing equipment; punching bags, body bags, a treadmill, a large array of weights, and assorted other training tools—some of which I was unfamiliar with. Right then, I was weighed and then told that they would like me to fight as a middleweight boxer. The gym also had a steam room, and a *steambox* (think rapid weight loss), together with the usual showers and locker room. There was everything that one might expect of a modern boxing club of that era.

Back in the manager's office, I was told that the club, if they liked what I showed them in the RING, would supply me with all I needed; shoes, socks and workout clothing including the special garb I would need for the regularly scheduled fights before the public. As a Golden Gloves boxer I would compete in the Ring in bouts of no more than three rounds, each lasting just three minutes. (Three minute rounds may not sound like much time for those who have never been in a *ring* fighting with a real boxing opponent, but trust me, you had better be in very good shape to last that long if you are to come out at the end of your round in one piece.) However, what finally really got my interest, persuading me to sign up, was that I would be given a stipend each time I fought in public, plus there would be a bonus amount above that, were I to win over my opponent. This intrigued me because I wanted to help out my parents by being as financially independent as possible, knowing that it was expensive to send my brothers and me so far away to school that year.

The very next afternoon, after school, I was back in the Club's gym getting assigned a locker, given training clothes, and being introduced to other boxers there, mainly with those about my weight category. Now my training went into full swing, a training manager observed and advised me while fellow boxers assisted. This was, of course, an entirely new, unique, and challenging culture, yet I got right into it. A light-heavyweight sparring partner, who I enjoyed working out with, and who was very helpful in training me, pointed out one of the other boxers who he said I should avoid getting in the ring with. This mean looking, heavier fighter got his perverted kicks, he said, by getting a new trainee in the ring, toying with him for a time, then callously and mercilessly beating on him awhile before knocking him out. Obviously, I had to watch myself carefully in this dangerous, violent *sport,* with a few of such unprincipled characters about.

Five nights a week I worked out at the '449' Club, honing my fighting skills, until one evening I was called into the office and told, "We now feel that you are learning our sport rapidly and are an asset to the

Club, so we would like to put you on the next Fight Ticket." This was a bit of a surprise to me. It had been less than a month since I had come aboard and, though I had been getting plenty of encouragement and positive feedback, I had no idea that I was really ready for this next big step. Calling Dad that night to see what he thought, he said to me, "Sammy, if your manager thinks you're ready for the Big Ring, then you probably are. You'll be fighting in your weight category, so there should ordinarily be no problem. I know that you will use your own good judgment, and that'll be enough for me. Just be sure to let your Mother and I know when you are scheduled and we'll be there to watch and cheer you on." Even my Parents were excited about this new sport, just as they had been when my brothers and I were playing football for our school.

My first big coming out fight had arrived, Tuesday, 21 February1950, 8:30 p.m., at the Shrine Mosque Auditorium in Springfield, Missouri. I had just turned 18 a month before, and had joined the Marine Reserves. It was a momentous time for me. That night's program listed the Fight Ticket as: SPRINGFIELD '449' CLUB—VS—ALGOA, (MO). The first six bouts listed on the program were for the lighter weight contenders. After an intermission the second half of the program featured the six heavier boxers' bouts, with mine listed second: SAMMY LARKIN: 160—VS—BOB LOYDE: 155.

That night the Club had dressed me out in dark blue trunks with a wide white strip down both sides, and thick heavy gloves, I was ready to go into the ring.

Was I nervous before my first public fight? You bet I was! Dad, Mom, and my two brothers were in the audience to watch me battle a slightly shorter broad shouldered foe from a local reform school, a real toughie.

In our workout room that fight-night, there were all kinds of people, much confusing loud talk, and many things going on—a whirlwind of activity. While I waited for my call (I saw none of the bouts), Jerry, my old trainer, took me off to one of our private side rooms and told me to lie down and rest on one of the massage tables, and gave me a soothing pre-bout rubdown and prep talk. He told me that we had plenty of time and he would come to get me when all was ready. Jittery and excited as I was, I somehow drifted off to sleep from nervous exhaustion.

The next thing I knew, Jerry, usually such an easy going fellow, was now all business; slapping me awake with a cold wet towel, and with clipped tones, instructing me as how to engage my opponent, all while taking me through crisp pre-bout exercises. A mandatory last minute pre-fight weigh-in was made, a shiny loose robe was draped over my shoulder, my gloves were laced on my fists, a cushioned tooth protector was shoved into my mouth, then I was hustled from that room into bright lights, the white hot center of a huge, and noisy, bloodthirsty sounding mob. The Ringmaster was calling out my name and statistics as I climbed through the ropes to my corner. I danced a couple of seconds, throwing straight punches in the empty air, hopefully showing poise and aggressiveness. My opponent stood shuffling his feet slightly on the other side of the ring, and just stared at me with an air of sheer disdain and disgust. My defining moment had arrived, I was finally on my way to *fame and glory* or to *the depths of defeat and gory.*

The referee called us boxers to the center of the ring, grasped each by a shoulder, and began a short list of preliminary cautions: "No hitting below the belt, break clean from a clinch when I tell you to, no head butting, go to a neutral corner when a man is down." Usually not much more than that was said, before closing with, "Now shake, then back off, and at the bell—come out fighting."

ROUND 1: Often the first round begins with the contestants moving about their opponent, tossing out punches to test and feel out their reactions, after which the real action begins in earnest. When our round began, however, my worthy opponent dove straight at my chest, head first, arms flailing wildly, looking for a body blow and a clinch. Wow! Obviously, this fearless kid was determined to bring the fight to me. Well, that was good for I had the longer arms, was quick, and could handle his rushes with punishing blows; this suited my style of fighting for the rest of the round.

ROUND 2: This round started out in a more classic style, with each of us throwing sharp left punches, following hopefully with a powerful and stinging right. The problem for me was that this stocky kid I was mixing it up with was a southpaw; his left hand was his power. Thankfully, my Coach had wised me for this, saving me from serious trouble with this dude, by teaching me techniques on how to counter this kind of fighter. The second round was full of lively action with blows thrown and connecting on both sides.

A panel of judges who gave points to the better style and effectiveness of the boxers scored our kind of boxing. Although I didn't know it, I was leading, taking both rounds on points. I thought I had barely been able to edge out my worthy opponent during the first six minutes of our bout,

ROUND 3: This last three-minute round could be the clincher for me, unless he knocked me unconscious. At this point, notwithstanding the positive encouragement I was receiving from Jerry in my corner, I was still not aware of my having the best point count. When the bell rang, it was now that the real fury of the fight began for both of us. It was our last chance. We were both now giving the contest everything we had, giving and receiving blow after blow, when suddenly my shorter opponent rushed in for a tight clinch and before the referee could break us apart, my opponent brought his head up in a sharp vicious BUTT to my face. Being just that much taller than he was, I was vulnerable to this illegal stratagem, and he certainly used this blow effectively.

Immediately, I was blinded and confused by a flood of blood streaming down and into my right eye from a three-month old wound that I had totally forgotten about. Seeing me half blind and backing off, this kid poured in with a flurry of blows to my face before the referee could temporarily stop the action.

Taken to my corner, I wasn't sure whether the fight was over or not. A doctor consulting with my worried

Coach, who was working swiftly to staunch the blood flow, determined that if the flow were stopped, then the round might continue for the next minute and a half, if I were willing (and I was.) I couldn't allow this cheating tough to win on a TKO. Now with the application of a thick coat of Vaseline over the cut, the remainder of our fight resumed, but unlike the first two rounds of the fight, when I had aggressively taken the fight to my opponent. Now I backed off a bit, obviously protecting myself so this aggressive kid—literally thirsting for my blood—could not get at my wounded eye. It was a furious conclusion to an exciting fight, till the final bell saved my eye from being busted open again. That last round went to the other fighter, but I had taken the first two rounds, and so won the fight.

I had won my first public boxing match, though bloody it was. Other fights I had, but this was the most dramatic and memorable. Of the several public fights that season, I lost not one and tied but one. At the end of the season, one of the managers proposed to take me north, to Chicago or Detroit to fight as a Middle Weight professional. Dad, when told of this proposal, wisely discouraged it, to his advice I agreed heartily. Why would I want to make a living getting my brain beat to mush? I had much more important plans for my future, for had I not already made up my mind to enter a Trappist monastery after graduating from high school.

In the Morning

In the morning
I look forward to the sun in the leaves of the
trees
Reflecting on blades of grass.
But more I seek the smile on your face,
and feel my arms enfolding you.

In the morning
I anticipate the day and the sharing time with
you,
touching your hair, and hearing you say "1 love
you."

In the morning
Of our lives,
all seems bright and promising,
exciting and eternal.
All is possible.

In the morning
we do not see the evening.
The shadows of life,
when that final day arrives.
Let the morning of your eyes
lead me lovingly into the night.

Marjory Bong-Ray Liu

Every workshop participant has interesting stories to tell, but none is more unusual or exciting than Marjory Liu's account of her life in China during and shortly after World War II.

In the workshops, we often discuss tone. Is the writing in narratives too emotional—or too coldly analytical? It seems to me that Marjory Liu has chosen exactly the right tone. Tone, of course, involves register or level of formality/ informality, but more than that, the author's involvement creates tone. Because Marjory Liu stands back from her personal history and tells us what happened, with few hints about her own emotional reactions, the tone is dispassionate and straightforward—which, it seems to me, is perfect. Marjory gives us the history and lets us infer the emotional impact that events must have had on her. The workshop colleagues agreed that Marjory's story would have been less effective if she had emoted. Her almost dispassionate objectivity was just right.

—W.R.W.

My Adventures in China During World War II

This narrative of events in my early life details how a few months after my April 1944 marriage to Dr. James Yu-ping Chen, in Japanese occupied Shanghai

91

during WWII, fate played its capricious hand, leading us to weather numerous adventures, beginning with our escape from Shanghai to Free China.

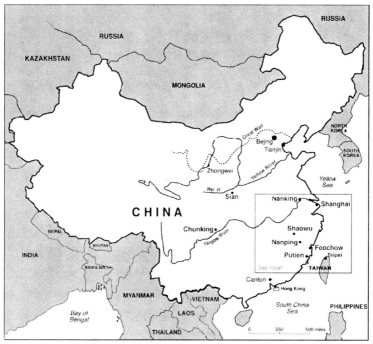

Map 1. China.

I was born in 1923, in Nanking (Nanjing today), the capital of China, and was named Marjory Liu, with my Chinese name of Pang-shui Liu (much later the spelling was legally changed to Bong-Ray Liu). My father, Ven-hai Liu, was Chinese, from Shensi (Shaanxi) province near Xian, by the Yellow River in northwest China. My mother, Annie Pickstock, hailed from Holmes Chapel, Cheshire in the English midlands. They met while fa-

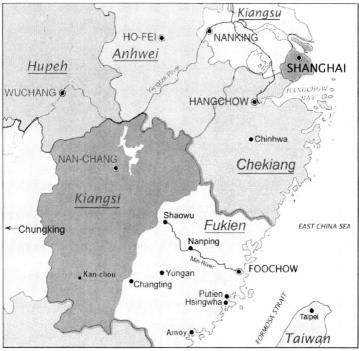

Map 2. Inset showing places involved in the trek.

ther was enrolled in a military academy in Cheshire. They married in London in 1914, while both were twenty years old, and then moved to China. At that time, East-West marriages were extremely rare, so my mother was a very courageous pioneer, to go to China, a strange far land, with my father. Years later they lived in Madison, Wisconsin, where father obtained his masters degree in political science and economics from the University of Wisconsin. Subsequently they returned to China. They had six children: four born in China, one in the U.S., and one in England.

When I was growing up in China, the country was greatly affected by the agonies and disruptions of wars on Chinese soil. There were civil wars, and warlord instigations (1920s–1949); the brutal Japanese occupation of Manchuria and parts of eastern China (1931–1945); World War II (1939–1945) and the Chinese Communist takeover in 1949. During many of those years my family and I had to evacuate our homes, face separation, and escape to safer areas in China. Decades of turmoil followed a century of uprisings and subjugation by territorial Western Powers, and then Japanese occupying Chinese territory. I went to school in many different places and finally spent my high school years in Shanghai in the 1940s.

During World War II, while living in Shanghai, I met James Yu-ping Chen M.D., when he came to our home to attend to my mother. I fell in love with my mother's handsome young physician, and eventually in April 1944 we married. Soon after our marriage, Jimmy and I decided to escape from Japanese occupied Shanghai to seek a life in Free China. Planning had been underway for some time as to the best escape method. We decided that traveling by sea, south to the port city of Foochow (Fuzhou), in Fukien (Fujian) province, would risk fewer encounters with the Japanese military. Jimmy's parents came from Foochow, and another young couple we knew that spoke the dialect of Foochow, elected to come with us. Our original plan was to sail to Foochow, but by the time our plans were set, Foochow had been taken over by Japanese forces. Therefore, we chose instead to go on to Putien (Putian), a port farther south, and from there, traverse an overland route west through the interior part of Fukien province. In early December of 1944, married only several months, we met the other couple on the dock in Shanghai, where a small sampan (sailboat) was waiting for us.

Instead of having the sampan to ourselves as had been agreed upon, there were over a dozen more men and women going with us. Although not the ideal situation, given the small size of the sampan and its limited accommodations, we decided it was now or never. We four went aboard, together with our heavy luggage.

We found that male passengers got deck space, while women, separated from their men, were stowed into a crawl-space cargo area set just below the main deck. Just four feet high, we women could only sit up, leaning back to back, or lie down next to each other, like canned sardines, in head to foot fashion. Incredibly, there was no toilet in the women's space, just a makeshift arrangement—a pail—for eight women and two babies. A few days into the voyage, human excrement made the stench unbearable. To make matters worse, in the dank darkness of our *cave,* we got soaked from rain leaking through from the deck. With only a limited outside view through a rectangular hatch hole cut into the wall of our prison, we felt trapped—as indeed we were. Only at night were women allowed to go up on deck to get a breath of fresh air. Passengers' heavy luggage was stored on deck, where the male passengers also spread their thin sleeping mattresses. With no cover overhead, men and luggage were exposed to the elements.

Fate intervened as soon as we sailed. What we didn't know then was that our voyage of supposedly three days would last much longer. Not long after we pulled anchor, our sampan stopped at the mouth of Shanghai harbor, and lay idle there for three days—the headwinds were not in our favor. During that tedious wait, we finished what little food and snacks we had managed to bring aboard. The captain claimed he could not go ashore to procure more food, even though our passage was supposed to include *room and board*. We were devastated—but what to do? We ended up pooling our cash and jewelry—even some wedding rings—in order to obtain some rice to eat. On the fourth day, we sailed out into the China Sea, looking forward to soon getting some decent food. Instead, all of us women and children, huddled together in our cramped storage space below deck, were given a large pail of watery rice porridge only once a day. Sometimes the gruel had fish or meat bones in it, from which the crew and male passengers had already picked off the flesh. Equally outrageous, only a limited amount of drinking water was allotted us women, and we were never, throughout the voyage, given water with which to bathe.

As if to make life more miserable, I developed dysentery. Weak, and continually hungry, I could rarely stomach any food. Most of the time I lay on my back, looking up at wet and slimy beams, where cockroaches (42—I had ample time to count them) were clinging. I was perpetually afraid that the cockroaches might lose their grip and drop onto our bodies. In retrospect, I don't know why nobody just plucked the cockroaches off, something I myself could never have dared to do. Many days it rained incessantly, so we had to contend with the leaks from the deck. We existed in a constant dampness, made worse by chilling winds that whistled through the open hatch in the wall.

We survived several storms at sea, when the pitching of our small sampan brought on bouts of crippling seasickness. During those storms; our drunk captain, incapacitated much of the time, left day-to-day control to the first mate. That did not stop the crazy captain however, when he was in a drunken stupor, from tossing our heaviest suitcases overboard one night—in order (he later testified) to lighten the load on the boat midst heaving storm waves.

It turned out that to gain speed, we had sailed way beyond the near-shore limit for small craft, and were far into the wide ocean where we saw gunboats, in the distance fortunately. We never did find out whether they were Chinese or Japanese. After seeing gunboats, and weathering storms, the captain wisely decided to avoid the high seas, and sailed closer to the very convoluted coastline of Chekiang (Zhejiang) and Fukien provinces.

One sunny morning, over one week after we had set sail, we sighted land, and thought we had reached Putien. However, that was wishful thinking. As we sailed into a harbor on a small island, we learned it was a pirate stronghold! I wondered, how could we have got lost, and landed in such dangerous waters?

As soon as the sampan docked, all the male passengers were ordered to line-up on deck to be inspected by the pirates. More cash and jewelry, hidden from the captain, were confiscated this time. All while we female passengers were huddled below deck, afraid to utter a sound. The two mothers kept their babies' mouths covered so their cries could not be heard. There was no telling what the pirates would do with so many women in hiding. My risk was even greater, because my Caucasian looks would bring suspicion as to why I was traveling freely, when all citizens of the Allies were in concentration camps near Shanghai. If I were to be held hostage, it would surely complicate matters for others. Thus, my throat was as dry as an empty water flask, while my heart was racing so fast, I thought it might jump out of my body! The pirates heard nothing from us women during their inspection—thank goodness! Thereafter, all their negotiations were held ashore, so we women felt safe for a while.

The pirates held our sampan in port for three days, during which time we were given our first decent meals since departing from Shanghai. Although we did not know it at the time, we learned later that our captain had actually been in league with the pirates, and some contraband items may have been exchanged in return for our safe passage the rest of the way at sea. Anyway, we sailed away and after four-more days reached Putien.

Immediately upon reaching shore, the four of us who had chartered the sampan, had the captain arrested, and put in jail for gross negligence and abusive behavior. He had had the audacity to renege on all our agreements. He failed to provide accommodations and food, drinking and bathing water; had dumped much of our luggage overboard, and he had not operated the boat in a safe manner. After being refunded part of our passenger fees, and feeling somewhat vindicated, we moved to Hsingwha (Xinghua), a nearby city, where we took a needed rest for a few days to be ready for the inland trek portion of our escape to western China.

In contrast to our sea voyage from Shanghai, we spent a quiet Christmas in Hsinghwa. I remember how peaceful it looked with its mostly ancient buildings and narrow streets, and the weather was balmy, much like southern California. Enjoying sunny skies and light breezes on Christmas day, we visited some historic sites. Hsinghwa, just north of Amoy, had a long history as the port of departure for many Chinese who for some centuries had emigrated across the straits of Formosa to the island of Taiwan (formerly Formosa). There they had assimilated with the former native Asians from the Pacific islands of Melanesia, and in modern days, considered themselves as Taiwanese.

Even though their dialect was difficult for me, we had delightful conversations with some of the adventurous, seagoing people of Hsinghwa. Most of all, we treasured our visit with Dr. Ke-hsin Li, a famous retired physician and a wonderfully talented artist. As he sat at a table with his painting materials spread out, we watched in amazement as he painted impromptu, three brush paintings of bamboo branches and plum blossoms using only black ink and red paint. As we marveled at the ease with which he wielded the large and small brushes, his masterful strokes transformed large blank pieces of rice paper into beautiful works of art. Dr. Li graciously gifted us with those lifelike paintings—treasures I have managed to preserve by being rolled into scrolls, all through the travails of wars and the rigors of travel. They still hang in my home as a reminder of our visit to Hsinghwa.

After Christmas, it was time to complete arrangements for our escape west over the mountains to Nanping in western Fukien province. We were strongly advised to obtain the guide services of two experienced police officers who knew the area and who would protect us well—for the right amount of money. We took the advice, blissfully unaware till halfway on our journey, our guides were known as police officers by day—robbers by night!

The mountainous region we were to cross was covered with subtropical foliage, with dark forests, where the overhead leaf-covered tree branches blocked sunlight, and where tangled shrubbery clotted the lower levels. Exotic plants and flowers bordered the jungle and its meandering paths. A spooky silence pervaded the area, and its eerie quiet seemed more menacing than any sounds. We seldom spoke, and then just in whispers as we stepped lightly in single file, led by our two security guides, with porters silently following us, safari-style, carrying what few worldly possessions we had left from our voyage, as well as extra clothing and food purchased in Hsinghwa. We all were edgy, alert to any hint of the presence of lurking tigers in the dense bush, because this was a habitat of the much-feared blue tiger—a ferocious animal known to kill and eat humans. Everyone was very cautious, taking care not to make any undue sound, not to talk nor even whisper. Never having heard of the blue tiger species, I didn't know what to expect, but I feared the consequences of any encounter.

It was dark when we finally reached the top of the mountain, and made camp on a patch of level ground surrounded by trees. We cooked our meal over a makeshift fire, and soon after, drifted fast asleep. I had hung up our clothes that needed drying, and placed some cooking utensils and other items on the ground. The following morning only one pot was missing, but I didn't mention it for I felt we were lucky not to have had anything else taken. Our *protection money* was well invested. We departed down the mountain on the west side, anxious to reach lower ground, and some indication of civilization where we would no longer need our police escorts. We never did encounter any blue tigers, although we had some scary moments when there were suspicious rustling sounds in the thick forest. When we finally reached a town on level ground, we said goodbye to our guides and porters, and boarded a bus bound for Nanping.

A hilly bustling market and college town, Nanping served as the mid-province crossroads of Fukien. Upon arriving there after a long bus ride, we were unable to find accommodations. The couple that accompanied us suggested we contact a relative of theirs. That relative had no room either, but they did offer us the use of a newly constructed barn intended for livestock that had grain stored temporarily inside. We thought of Joseph and Mary when they were forced to stay in an animal stall. However, we jumped at the chance, and for a few nights, slept comfortably under cozy quilts, on cots woven from pliable, yet strong, freshly peeled slivers stripped from bamboo trunks. We could have done much worse.

We were in bamboo country. In this region, like the versatile peanut, bamboo had many uses. People ate tender bamboo shoots, grew bamboo plants in pots to decorate the home and courtyard, made all kinds of bamboo furniture—tables, chairs, stools, beds, wardrobes, cabinets, and even cooking utensils—pots and pans, lids, ladles, containers, chopsticks, forks, spoons and the like. Most amazing was the way bamboo was used to build complete houses—in an incredibly short time—I saw the bamboo grow over a foot in one night. Even when as tall as a tree, bamboo sways in a wind or storm, but never breaks. I was reminded of the Taoist saying; that if rigid—one breaks, but if pliant—one adapts and endures.

We had reached Nanping during the school winter break, which gave us enough time to find temporary jobs before venturing further inland. I accepted a position teaching music at Nanping Women's College and taught English and music at the adjacent Jienping High School. Jimmy shared a medical office with another physician. We thought our living situation would remain stable for a while, and indeed things were going well, until mid-semester. Our lives were suddenly disturbed by a tremendous high-school student strike. The students were frenzied over some altercation between northern and southern Fukienese students. They wanted to get the principal to settle the matter—the mood was ominous.

One evening, we were just sitting down to supper in our apartment provided by the school, when suddenly we were interrupted by loud thumping sounds in the hallway, like a thundering herd of cattle. When our door was pounded, we opened it to the yelling of these rebellious students, angrily shouting "Hao Dong, Hao Dong"—meaning "Principal, Principal!" They thought he was living in our building, and might even be hiding in our place, so they brushed us aside and tramped through our apartment looking for the poor man. As soon as they discovered he was not in our place, they stampeded out the door and continued further along the hallway, their heavy boots clattering and then fading into the distance.

Jimmy and I were struck silent by this sudden intrusion, and we wondered whether all students in Fukien were this hotheaded and uncontrollable. Afterwards, we learned that a truce had been reached between the two feuding student groups, and the principal remained as principal. After that incident, things stayed relatively quiet for the rest of the semester. I managed to prepare and produce two spring musical concerts, one with college students, and one at the high school. Both were quite successful, so everyone was happy, and looked forward to more musical programs.

However, after the end of the spring semester, Jimmy wanted to move further inland toward our final destination—Chungking (Chongqing) in west China.

So I left the schools and Jimmy his practice, then we traveled south to Yungan (Yongan), the wartime capital of Fukien province, where my father lived and had his offices, and where my brother Raymond was working.

When we arrived at Father's house, he asked to see me alone upstairs, where he showed displeasure at my having married a poor doctor rather than some high-placed government official. Later, at Father's request, Jimmy came upstairs, and they engaged in a cold, polite exchange of pleasantries. As Jimmy and I were preparing to depart, Father suddenly announced, "I would like to hold a banquet for you tomorrow before you leave Yungan." Well, the banquet took place, and if I remember correctly, Raymond was also present, but most of the other guests were Father's working staff. I got the impression that this whole event was a mere formality. He was only putting on a show of *doing the right thing,* not as a parent, but as a person in his position as Director of the Bureau of Audit in Fukien province, so he would not *lose face* among his associates and superiors.

Raymond confided to me later that Father hated Fukienese people in general, because he found many of them to be conniving, shifty, and unreliable. That may have been the reason he was unjustly prejudiced to anyone from Fukien, and especially Foochow. This was ironic since his only married children both had spouses from Foochow—Raymond's wife, Linda, and my husband Jimmy. Father sealed his disapproval of my marriage by refusing to give me any wedding present, even though it was customary for all Chinese parents to do so. Full of disappointment and sadness, to distance ourselves from Father, and to continue our escape to Free China, we moved south to Changting (Changding).

Changting had an airfield that provided a way out to Chungking, the WWII capital of Free China. We stayed in Changting in case there was a plane available to fly us to Chungking. While waiting, we spent time getting to know some of the locals and travelers moving in and out of the city, including US Air Force personnel.

Jimmy had been a consultant at Shenghwa Pharmaceutical Company in Shanghai, one of the largest in China at that time. They had branches in several cities in Free China, one of which was in Changting, and so Shenghwa managers befriended us, and gave us a room within their offices in which to stay. The company manager was very religious, and he held evangelical Christian services outside our room several times a week. It seemed rather strange to have this activity in a small outpost in the hinterlands of Fukien, where *any* Christian presence would be unlikely.

The workers at Shenghwa heard Jimmy call me Marjory, but to them the name sounded like Ma-zwei, which meant *horse's mouth* in their dialect, and so they would laugh every time they heard it. (It was a good thing my name didn't translate into a horse's behind—that would have been no laughing matter!) Of course, in parts north, Marjory was pronounced Ma-ji, which was identical in sound to *horse & chicken;* either way, Chinese folk must have thought my parents lovers of animals in order to give me such a name.

Among the steady stream of visitors in Changting were American Air Force personnel who, since Pearl Harbor was bombed in 1941, had use of the local airfield for flights in and out of China. Many were with General Chenault's Flying Tigers, who flew over the *Hump* from Burma, carrying wartime military supplies to the Chinese Nationalists. Because of my Caucasian looks, I was considered an anomaly among other Chinese, but the American airmen were friendly, yet respectful.

I had important things on my mind, of course. Every day we inquired about flights going west, yet nothing materialized. Finally, after a month, there came word that a seat was available—for Jimmy only. He was designated to carry a supply of ephedrine (Mahuang), a drug that was to be used for the war effort, to keep the Nationalist pilots awake on their dangerous flight missions. Ephedrine was most scarce at that time, and was produced only in small quantities by pharmaceutical companies. (Currently ephedrine is the banned ingredient for many diet pills in U.S.A. because of its dangerous effects.)

Unfortunately, I was specifically prohibited from leaving with Jimmy due to an unfortunate incident that had occurred just prior to our arrival in Chanting. Fate perhaps, but a plane carrying several men and one woman passenger had trouble in the air, and everyone aboard was ordered to parachute out of the plane. The woman, however, was in a panic, and refused to jump out. The pilot, like a ship's captain, would not abandon the plane until everyone aboard had departed, so he stayed with the woman—they died when the plane crashed and blew up in flames. Because of this fateful tragedy, women were no longer allowed to ride in a plane. I knew the importance of Jimmy's mission and so, very reluctantly agreed that he should go and I would find a way to join him later.

As newlyweds, we were worried as to when we would meet again. Nevertheless, Jimmy was excited about contributing to the war effort after being unable to help while in Japanese-occupied Shanghai since 1942. Therefore, I held back my tears and tried to sound optimistic when I bade him goodbye at the Changting airport on the morning of August 10, 1945.

I shall remember that day forever, because that very same afternoon (I later learned) when Jimmy stepped out of his plane in Chungking, there were great masses of people shouting and dancing, and fireworks were going off. Jimmy told me that he had thought: What a huge reception just to welcome our plane landing safely. Then someone nearby yelled, "The war is over, the war is over: Japan has surrendered—after eight long years!" News had spread quickly that two American atom bombs had decimated the cities of Hiroshima and Nagasaki, on August 6 and 9, forcing the surrender of Japan on August 10, which became official on August 15.

In Changting, when I heard the news that the long war between the Japanese and the Chinese had finally ended, I was both tremendously elated and relieved beyond measure. I was, however, also devastated, that by a stroke of fate, the day that Jimmy left for Chungking was the same day the war ended. All our efforts seemed so wasted, so in vain—just a few hours later and there would have been no need for Jimmy to go—we would have still been together. I was overwhelmed. I could not internalize the irony; our years of waiting in Shanghai to escape to free China; our treacherous journey by both sea and land; our months of waiting to fly west to the wartime capital of Chungking; was all for nothing. For the first time I felt truly alone, no husband, no family, no real friends, and no clear way of returning to my home in Shanghai. Jimmy's co-workers at Shenghwa, understanding my predicament, were very kind to me, and generously offered to help me with temporary lodging and some money to get by.

Then came word that Miss Phoebe Wei, former head of the music department at Nanping Women's College where I had taught the previous semester, was looking for me. She had accepted a similar position at Fukien Christian University (F.C.U.) in Shaowu, and she wanted me to join her in the music department. I had no idea how she had located me. I felt blessed that just at that crucial moment, when I had no firm idea of what to do next, here was the solution to my problem.

During those postwar weeks, private communications between Chungking and Changting were impossible, for the airwaves were jammed with both military and civilians trying to get in touch with their families. I sent several telegrams to Jimmy, but never received any reply, so I despaired of hearing from him anytime soon. I knew I had no immediate hope of being able to get home to Shanghai, for all means of transport had been commandeered by people with influence. Consequently, I decided that until things returned to normal, I would accept the offer to teach at F.C.U. in Shaowu for at least a semester. By then, Jimmy might have been able to get to Shanghai to meet me there, so with that hope in mind I left for F.C.U.

Many leading universities had chosen to move away from the eastern coastal cities to sites further inland where their students could study in peace without fear of Japanese takeovers. Among them was F.C.U.; they had moved from Foochow on the east coast of Fukien, inland to Shaowu in the foothills of northwestern Fukien province. Much of Fukien was away from the main trade routes as the hilly terrain, ill-kept roads, and lack of railroads made transportation difficult, which was precisely why Shaowu, a small town at a tributary of the Min River that flowed all the way down to the coast, was selected as the wartime campus of F.C.U. The site was further northwest of Nanping, the college town where my husband, Jimmy, and I had stayed for half a year after our escape from Shanghai in late 1944. So I moved to Shaowu in the fall of 1945, to teach in the music department.

Educational materials were scarce when I joined the Shaowu faculty in the fall of 1945, right after WWII ended. The students, several hundred strong, were strapped for even paper and pencils. Therefore, the enterprising students made their own paper from pulp ground from thin slivers of bamboo. Their small makeshift printing press churned out daily newsletters and syllabi, and sometimes concert programs as well as music scores were laboriously copied by hand and then printed. Nevertheless, the school spirit overall was high as students thought of themselves as adventurers and pioneers in the quest for higher learning.

I was assigned a one-bedroom brick row house with a courtyard in front. I cooked my own food, or sometimes ate in the school cafeteria. Food in that isolated region was rather scarce because there were few local crops, and it was difficult to import much other than staples. Even rice was hard to acquire, let alone meat of any kind. The students had a sparse diet, but they never complained, since everyone there was in the same situation.

As I became more acquainted with the students, especially those in my own classes, I grew more and more sympathetic at their attempts to pursue university degrees in the face of most trying circumstances. Many sacrificed a great deal in coming to Shaowu, leaving behind families, homes, and friends. I would occasionally invite them as a group over to tea, and decided to celebrate the Autumn Moon Festival with them. I bought several large sacks of fresh taro root (similar to yams) from a market in town, cooked them in huge vats over an open fire on the hillside, mashed them up and added lots of brown sugar. I served steaming bowls of sweet taro pudding to the students, who gratefully devoured this treat. Afterwards, as was the custom in China, in the light of the full moon we sang songs. Mostly old, in English, well-known favorites of these young Western influenced students, such as, *Beautiful Dreamer, Old Black Joe, Suwanee River, and Let Me*

Call You Sweetheart. It was an enjoyable evening, and it served as respite from the harsh realities of daily existence in remote Shaowu, and from my unanticipated separation from Jimmy.

Chinese students throughout the 20th century spearheaded many movements, primarily educational and political protests. I did not think that the sleepy little town of Shaowu would see any uprisings, but I was mistaken, for it seemed as though the student strike while I was in Nanping four months earlier, was being repeated. This time the university students declared a strike about providing a social room where coeds could meet outside of classes. The university, claiming lack of space, initially denied their request, so these hotheaded Fukienese students staged a sit-down, effectively barring anyone from attending major classes.

The student strike ended when the university provided a public social room on campus, then everything appeared to return to normalcy. Again, I was wrong, because a sinister event with dire consequences occurred towards the end of the fall semester. The whole region was suddenly struck with bubonic plague, a most uncommon incident in that part of China. It started when a janitor at the university died, and the next day, a student also succumbed to this dreaded disease. No one had anticipated this, so there was no medicine available to combat the plague. The only preventative measure available was to dust one's living quarters with lime powder, a strong disinfectant.

Even as more and more people were infected and more houses were dusted with lime, I foolishly rejected any offer to do likewise, simply because the powder's overpowering odor caused me to gag and choke. I went about my classes as usual, even with steadily dwindling student attendance. Although students fled the campus en-masse to avoid infection and probable death, I still refused to think that anything would happen to me. Only when I found a huge dead rat in my own courtyard, on its back, its four legs pointed up to the sky, did I hurriedly get some lime powder and dust my own living quarters.

By then the campus was deserted, and with few signs of life, was as quiet as a graveyard. I had never seen such a mass exodus happen in just a few days, and it brought home to me the severity of the situation. Few students stayed, and all classes were suspended for the rest of the semester. As one by one the faculty and staff left, and only a handful remained, I was finally persuaded to leave Shaowu by boat, the only means of transportation left. Bringing just a few belongings, I joined five or six others in a small, open, motored junk down the Min River. Our destination was Foochow on the east coast and site of the original campus of F.C.U., and we expected to land there in a few days.

With cramped space in the junk, our group of both teachers and students had little to do but take turns to stand and stretch our legs, eat cold meals, sleep fitfully, and talk to pass the time. I remember we had interesting discussions about many things, but these were all discontinued when we approached rapids. We soon were dismayed to learn our captain and his assistant had no special means to prevent the junk from capsizing as it dipped and wallowed through the turbulent sections, nor did they have lifejackets for us. Many times, we felt our lives were in extreme danger as the small junk was tossed about like a toy in the swirling waters. When we encountered several such rapids in succession, I was petrified with fear, my heart pounding so furiously, I fully expected it to jump out of my body! Yet, all we could do was to grip tightly to the junk, and pray. Somehow, fate intervened, because we all survived. Between rapids, there were relaxing stretches of quiet waters. By nightfall, we were thankful to find a place to sleep onshore.

The next morning we resumed our journey, and everything was peaceful until late afternoon, when the captain and his young assistant in the makeshift galley were preparing food. Suddenly, there was loud shouting as two pairs of bare feet slapped along the narrow gunwale of the junk. The gunwale was a ledge only a few inches wide, yet there was the furious captain, waving a huge chopping knife, chasing his assistant along the ledge, round and round the junk, causing it to tilt from side to side, the captain all the while was shouting obscenities. The poor assistant was trying to avoid being butchered alive, while we passengers were struck dumb with disbelief. It all happened so quickly, it was hard for us to react, but finally someone yelled for the captain to desist and to calm down. It apparently worked. Perhaps not wanting to lose his paying passengers, the captain went back to preparing the meal. Whew!

We passengers, however, could not relax after all that excitement. How could I have ever imagined encountering another crazy captain, after the one on the sampan that carried us to Putien—the drunken captain who had tossed our luggage overboard during a storm, and had led us into a pirate stronghold? Yet again, I was at the mercy of another drunkard of a captain as the junk swerved and swayed with no one at the helm. When we docked that night and went ashore, we made sure we would never engage that captain again. The next morning, we secured the services of a new and saner captain, and all went well as we ended our trip downstream, and reached the beautiful city of Foochow at sunset.

After arriving in Foochow, my only thought was how to return to Shanghai and meet up with my husband. I still had not heard from Jimmy for over half a year and I was desperate to join him and get on with our lives. Flying was the quickest way, so I arranged a flight out of Foochow. I was told that I could not take any luggage so, came the morning of the flight, I appeared at the airport looking like an overstuffed scarecrow. I was wearing three or four layers of pants and tops, my arms hung straight out because the clothing was so thick I could hardly bend my elbows. I had all the clothes I owned right on my back, and I carried only a small bag of essentials with me. Imagine my surprise and disappointment when I learned I had been bumped off, for my seat was given instead to someone with a higher priority: That meant I could not fly that day, nor, I suspected, was it going to be easier at a later date. Therefore, I gave up on flying home and turned to Plan B.

That plan was to go by sea again, traveling the reverse of the route Jimmy and I took when we escaped from Shanghai. Nothing should go wrong, I thought, since I would be on a commercial ship traveling a well-known sea route. As fate would have it, I arrived at the dock in the afternoon at the appointed time, to be told that the ship had already departed that morning. What a frustration! I railed long at why I had not been told of the change, until I learned a few days later that the ship, carrying over a hundred passengers, had struck an old Japanese-laid mine in the Shanghai harbor, and all except two people had perished! I then strongly felt that my life having been saved so many times was for a purpose. Even so, I was to spend much of the remainder of my life wondering why I was so fortunate when many others had lost their lives. I was now faced with Plan C, going overland to Shanghai.

I remember starting this journey going north by bus from Foochow, till the bus broke down in the middle of nowhere. Another passenger and I decided to walk, and so we plodded onward. We were on a desolate country road when it started to grow dark; there were no buildings in sight, other than a pigsty. We hurried there and gathered some straw on which to lie down and rest our weary heads for the night. Surrounded by sleeping pigs, we were too tired to care, and managed a night of fitful sleep. The next morning we resumed walking until we arrived at a small town. That's when my companion decided not to go any further; determined, I then pressed on, alone.

Farther on, I managed to arrange a ride in a covered truck that was heading north. I sat next to the driver, and all was well until we climbed into some hills and the truck began to sway from side to side. I thought that was rather odd, but ignored it, until suddenly, the truck zigged where it should have zagged and went off the road. It rolled over and over several times going down a steep embankment. It happened so quickly I had no time to be afraid, but again, as luck, or fate, would have it, we landed right side up, and all I sustained were some rather deep bruises and sprains.

The truck driver got out, went to the back of the truck and opened the rear door. Much to my horror, I saw a dozen or more people stumble out, in various stages of pain and fright. The driver said they had been locked inside to prevent them from falling out. They were so shook up and battered from the truck rolling over and over down the hill, that I am sure many of them needed medical treatment. I don't know what became of them, but while the driver was waiting for help, and knowing that I could not assist them, I resolved to move on so that I would not get jinxed or jinx anybody else with my fateful close encounters with so many disasters.

Several miles farther along, I reached a railroad station. I was able to negotiate a ride in an open railcar that had been used to transport smelly cattle. There were many others also standing, crammed into this one railcar for the long journey. When it began to rain, we all got soaked with no recourse but to tough it out until we reached our destination—the lake city of Hangchow.

I recalled a family friend who lived in Hangchow so, as a forlorn and bedraggled refugee on his doorstep, he was kind enough to take me in. For the first time in a long while, I enjoyed a nice hot bath and changed into clean clothes, then promptly fell asleep from the exhaustion of my long and eventful journey.

The next night, my host and his family treated me to a lovely banquet. I enjoyed every dish, until they unveiled the piéce de resistance—jumping grasshoppers! Although the grasshoppers had been lightly stir-fried, there were still some hardy critters twitching on the platter. As the guest of honor, I was expected to be the first to enjoy this *delicacy*. Regardless, I just couldn't bring myself to put this live insect into my mouth. As a polite gesture, I did manage, gingerly, to land one on my plate, where it writhed and wiggled for some time before expiring. I still cringe when I think of it, but am glad to say I have never been *treated* to a similar experience.

Since I had lived in Hangchow in 1936–37, and had loved taking walks around West Lake, a beautiful serene body of water divided by a causeway into two lakes, I looked forward to visiting some of my old haunts. However, the quiet, peaceful, and lovely picture-book setting of Hangchow did not inspire the atmosphere and mood enjoyed on earlier visits. Maybe it was because I was anxious to return to Shanghai, and so I was relieved when at last I was able to travel the last leg of my return trip to Shanghai, aboard a passenger train.

I arrived in Shanghai late at night, and found the streets deserted, which was unusual for even the dark and cold of early spring. For some reason, I had a feeling of foreboding, of alienation. I did not feel at home any-more, even though I had lived in Shanghai for six years during my teens, until escaping with Jimmy to Free China in 1944. I mused, perhaps one cannot return home from a long absence and expect everything to be as before, largely because we ourselves have changed.

I hired a pedicab (a three-wheeled open air cab driven by a bicyclist) for the long ride home across town. When Jimmy's family saw me at their front door, they were totally surprised, but unlike at my father's home in Yungan, they warmly welcomed me and made me feel at home. Welcomes aside, upon inquiring as to Jimmy's whereabouts, I was told, that just a few days earlier, he had boarded a former U.S. troop ship for San Francisco. The news shattered me. I suddenly felt completely drained, emotionally and physically, and wondered if fate would ever allow Jimmy and me to be together again.

In Shanghai, I saw a few of my old friends but, as in Hangchow, I felt out of place and had feelings that were hard to share with others. Money was a constant worry because I had never received any from Jimmy at any time, so I had to inquire around as to any paying jobs for me to handle. In post-war Shanghai, UNRRA (United Nations Relief and Rehabilitation Association) was a good instance of Sino-American cooperation. The

Chinese arm of UNRRA was CNRRA and its office was near to UNRRA's. I got a job at CNRRA as an office assistant, where I did typewriting, took shorthand, and filed masses of governmental documents. The job made me quite familiar with the socio-economic problems in the aftermath of war-torn China. At the same time I was trying to find a way to join Jimmy in San Francisco.

After following several blind leads for getting exit permits from Shanghai to go abroad, I realized that bureaucratic red tape was holding me back. Knowing that, I decided to go to the source. That was why I traveled on my own from Shanghai to Nanking, the capital, where all the governmental bureaus still operated, and where I would find out how to expedite my permit approval. Accordingly, I marched into the Foreign Ministry knowing nobody and armed only with two recommendation letters.

To an agent at the front desk, I stated my request for a Chinese Nationalist passport in order to join my husband in the USA. As luck, or fate, would have it, the agent read my Chinese name, (spelled at that time) Liu Pang-shui, and asked me, "Do you know Liu Pang-chen?"

I exclaimed "Why . . . Yes! He's my eldest brother, Raymond. How do you know him?"

He replied with much enthusiasm, "We were schoolmates here in Ginling Middle School, and I got to know him well!" Following this revelation he did all he could to assist me in filling out the forms, and I received a brand new passport—that day! I felt as if I had won a lottery. I was so happy to have succeeded where many others had to wait for months and even years to obtain passports. I went back to Shanghai, dancing on air, armed with increased hope and bustling confidence, hoping that the next step of acquiring an American visa would be soon accomplished.

Prior to my visa application, I had been accepted as an AAUW (American Association of University Women) scholarship recipient to study at Julliard School of Music in New York City, from which my former piano instructor, Mrs. Kwouk at St. Mary's Hall, had graduated many years earlier. However, the final acceptance papers for the scholarship were delayed, and knowing that a student visa would take still longer to obtain, I decided that the visitor's visa would get me to the U.S. sooner. I was anxious to leave because there were still unresolved issues between the Nationalist government of Chiang Kai-shek and Mao Tse-tung's Communists. The situation was most volatile and unpredictable. However, it took over a year for my US visa to be processed, and when I got it, it was only a visitor's visa, good for just six months in the USA.

It was in 1947, just a year after I had started working at CNRRA, that I was able to leave Shanghai for San Francisco, where Jimmy was affiliated with the University of California Medical School. My older sister, Barbara, and my second oldest brother, John, accompanied me on the former troop ship, General Meigs. They were assigned to different quarters than me. As a Chinese national, I was put in quarters for Chinese. I was given a top bunk in a cavernous space full of four-tiered bunks. Inches above me were not cockroaches, as in my 1944 sampan escape from Shanghai, but steam pipes that ran the whole length of the ceiling. During the entire voyage of about two weeks, I sweltered under those pipes, even when suffering terribly with seasickness. I was only able to eat watery rice porridge, made by a contingent of Chinese passengers on board.

I will never forget my first glimpse of America, as our ship approached San Francisco Bay in the early morning. From the wide expanse of blue ocean, a shoreline appeared and then tall buildings seemed to rise out of the mist, beckoning us to a new world and a new life. I gazed in wonderment as we sailed nearer and nearer, everyone around me excited yet silent, until we reached the dock. Then pandemonium. Everybody yelled and ran back and forth for a time, then calmed down, waiting eagerly for instructions to disembark.

My joy at coming to *The Land of the Free* was tempered by my first taste of racial discrimination. It was when the passengers were segregated according to race or nationality, not by names alphabetically or by family. Thus, Barbara who had been born in the USA and therefore an American citizen was allowed to leave the ship that first day. The next day, John who had been born in England, went ashore. Since I had been born in China, it was only on the third day that I was finally allowed to leave with the others of Chinese citizenship. Poor Jimmy! He came all three days to the ship's dock to wait for me to disembark in vain, until the third day.

We had a tearful reunion. Jimmy didn't know what to say and I was choked with emotion. We were finally together after two years of separation, having endured all sorts of hardships. We never anticipated that new-lyweds would have to experience such setbacks, caused by the events of war. However, all our misadventures were forgotten when we met again on the docks of San Francisco in 1947. Deeply thankful this glad day had come, and that we were both safe and healthy, we looked forward to living the rest of our lives in peace in the U.S.A.

QI (Chee) *

Qi, the necessary ingredient of life,
Yet evanescent and in changing garb.
The essence of ourselves we take for granted,
Without which we are robbed of existence.
The fashionable byword of pseudo-mystics,
Who flaunt their qi and market it as gurus.
This wordless *It* that's not for sale,
Where seeking defeats and being attains.
This vital rhythm which sets our pace,
Whose melody is the high and low of our days.
Description defies, for understanding is mute—
—No sparks and levitation,
No tongues and gibberish,
No gimmicks or easy path;
Our only proof an inner clarity and power,
Constant and true, open and radiant.
We can then know without learning,

We can love without trying,
We can live beyond dying . . .
For infinity as qi resides within us all!

*Qi, pronounced Ch'i or Chee, a Chinese word for breath, breath of life, air, vitality, fundamental energy of the universe.

Snow in Beijing

My first snow in Beijing—I taste its silent hue.
The world a downy sheen
Of flakes and stars, and I . . .
Enveloped in its vastness,
Mute with wonder and with joy. . . .
If only my pen danced poetry,
You'd hear the song in my heart!

To Ai Ching, a leading twentieth-century Chinese poet in Beijing, whose pen danced poetry.

Kathy Recupero

The past—reliving it, recapturing it, reconstructing it. That's an opportunity that the workshops afford participants. Why, one might ask, do folks need a workshop in order to record their pasts? The answer is twofold: exigency and audience. Participants know that they must produce some work each week—or feel guilty; they've committed themselves, and they must fulfill that commitment. Furthermore, they're not writing diaries with themselves as the sole audiences; they are writing for audiences, for readers who will respond to their work. Another factor is community. Workshop participants feel that they are members of a community and that their colleagues want to read what they have written and respond to it.

Kathy Recupero's writings are perfect examples of personal diary entries that have been transformed into memoirs for a broad readership.

—W.R.W.

As I Remember It—Love at First Slight

This is the way I remember it. In 1961, I was a sophomore at College of the Holy Names, a women's private college in Oakland, California. In September, it was traditional to have a *Co-Rec Day* with Saint Mary's of California, the local men's college, where we joined in sports, picnicking, sitting around socializing, and ending the day with a dance after dinner. We girls always looked forward to the event, discussing for several days what we would wear and who we wanted to *hustle*— the word of choice in the sixties—meaning *flirt with,* hoping to get asked out on a date.

That day I was walking on campus with my girl-friend, Katie, and I said to her, "There's a guy I would sure like to meet." She spied two fellows walking along in front of us, one short, dark, and stocky, and the other tall, blond, and slimmer.

Assuming I meant the tall blond guy, she said, "Oh, I know his name. It's Bart." Actually, I was looking at the shorter one; I liked his self-assured walk; his build, how he laughed and talked animatedly. He just looked like a fun guy with character; not super handsome.

Later that night at the dance while "twisting the night away," *he* noticed me and asked me to dance. I was having a great time getting to know him when, while he was talking, the piece of gum he was chewing fell out of his mouth, he bent down, picked it up, and without pausing, put it back in his mouth. It was so disgusting that he lost his appeal to me. In his defense, the guys had been drinking beer all day, normal for Co-Rec Day; I may have had a couple myself. But no excuse.

About a month later, Sergeant Shriver came to my college one evening, to introduce the Peace Corps. Being interested, I went down from the dorm to the meeting, which was held in one of the classrooms. Some of the guys from the men's college also attended, and I saw *him* again. There he was and I couldn't keep my eyes off him. He was with a bunch of guys and as he was leaving, coming down the aisle where he was going to pass me, I casually "bumped" into him and said, excuse me, like I hadn't noticed him. He remembered me but not my name. We walked outside together talking about the new Peace Corps, and he eventually said, "Would you go out with me if I asked you?"

"Well, maybe . . ." I said. You know, playing it cool.

I turned at the corner to our dorm, and it being dark, hiked up my skirt and took three flights of stairs, two steps at a time, to run and tell my roommate that Dave Recupero was going to ask me out! I was ecstatic. Only ten years later, did he tell me that he had followed me around the corner, and saw me run up those stairs.

Well, I waited by the phone expecting him to call the next night, and then the next night, and then, for sure, the next night. It turned out to be February 22, 1962, five months later, when he finally called to ask me to a basketball game. Agreeing to go, I had no idea that we were going to just listen on the radio with a bunch of other people, to his college team playing an out of town game. As I later found out, the guys were excited because it was the first radio broadcast of a live game, for a game being played with Loyola down south. Not being a real basketball fan, this was not an exciting first date for me. It did pick up later, however, when we joined his roommate and his girlfriend, Judy, whom I knew from my college, to go for coffee. I did let him kiss me good night, which was a little racy on a first date in those days, but he was a good kisser.

Later in the week, I ran into Judy at school and told her that I really had a good time with Dave and was hoping that he would call me back. She told her boyfriend who told Dave that I would like to date him again. Dave reportedly said that he was surprised because he didn't have that good a time and that I wasn't a very good kisser, but maybe he'd give me another chance.

We continued to date every weekend after that, until a couple months later, I realized that we were dating every Saturday night, but what was happening on Friday nights? Well, it turned out he had a standing Friday night date also . . . with Monique, a cheap, bleached-blond hussy, probably from a *public* school, if you want to know what I thought. She must have been a better kisser? When I gained more confidence I gave him the ultimatum: her or me.

That is how I remember it . . . 45 years later.

Daddy, a Beloved Irishman

Daddy is John Maury Faherty (aka Jack or Jackson) born December 9, 1908 in Memphis, Tennessee, the youngest of four children; two brothers and one sister, Francis, Michael and Jeanette (who died young before Daddy was born). His father, Michael William Faherty, was an engineer who traveled the country, selling pipe fitting equipment to oil companies. His mother was Minnie O'Donnell, a homemaker, who died when Daddy was about nine. When we asked him what his mother died from, Daddy would say that he didn't know, just that his mother was in bed a lot, got weaker and weaker, and died. He remembered climbing up on her bed often to talk with her. We surmised that she had a disease like tuberculosis or cancer.

After Daddy's mother died, his father, Michael, inherited the total care of his three sons, enrolling them in boarding school at Spring Hill College in Mobile, Alabama. Spring Hill was the first Catholic college in the Southeast, the third oldest Jesuit college in the country, and the fifth oldest Catholic college in America. The priests also ran a high school on the campus, and agreed to accept John as a student, young as he was, to keep the brothers together. They taught him separately until he reached high school age, and joined his older brothers. He graduated from Catholic High School in Memphis. He was partially raised by his favorite aunts, Ceil and Kate O'Donnell, sisters who lived at 1600 Vance Avenue in Memphis. He talked so fondly of them while my five siblings and I were growing up that we felt like we knew them, we even had their address memorized, but never visited there. I think the aunts did visit California once.

After graduation from high school in 1926, Daddy went off to Santa Clara University in California. His father lived in Van Nuys then, and his older brothers were married, one living in Tennessee, the other in Texas. He thrived in college and often talked about his many friends and experiences there. Daddy graduated in 1930, and he loved to tell us that Andy Devine was a classmate of his.

His first job out of college was as a teller for Security-First National Bank in Los Angeles, while living in Van Nuys. He eventually changed to Bank of America at Wilshire and La Brea in Los Angeles, and worked there until 1952.

He met Mother on a blind date at a beach party around 1934 when she was 18 years old. The eight year difference in ages seemed to be no hindrance to their life together. They had their ups and downs, but I don't think age was a factor. They married on November 11, 1937 in St. Victor's Church in Hollywood, where Mother grew up. She actually was a parishioner of Blessed Sacrament Church, but she was shy and terrified of walking up the long aisle in that large church.

After their marriage, they moved into one of the rental houses in Hollywood owned by Mother's family, where their first child, Eileen, was born in 1939. In 1941, they bought their own three-bedroom house, at 1502 Genesee Avenue in Los Angeles, where Mr. Faherty (my grandfather) lived with them for a short time, before he died in 1942. Several years after Daddy died, we found a diary of his dated 1941, in which he wrote that if the owners accepted his offer of $1,500 he would go to daily Mass for a year. Knowing Daddy, I'm sure he did go to daily Mass, since he never fell back on a promise. That same year, Mother had a second child, their son Michael, who died from a defective heart, or *blue baby*, when he was three days old.

Joy came back into their hearts, I'm sure, when I was born in October 1942, but this story is not about me. Mary Ann was born in 1945, Tom in 1947, Joan in 1951 and Sheila in 1954. Sometime during those years Daddy's spinster cousin, Loretta Griffin, came to live with us. When Tom was born, Mother told her they needed the room for their fourth child. After the fifth child was born, they decided that we needed to move into a larger house, and in December 1952, we moved to San Marino, California, into a four-bedroom home where Mother and Daddy lived out the rest of their lives.

When they moved to San Marino, Daddy studied for his contractor's license and after passing the test, started building custom homes. He built homes in Tarzana, Glendora, and San Gabriel. He was not known as a workaholic, but rather as the congenial Irishman who loved to host a party. He loved people, and often on a Sunday morning, he would run into friends at Mass and invite them for dinner that same evening— without conferring with Mother. Mother did all the work, as I never remember Daddy going to the market or helping to prepare the meal. Probably Mother never asked him. It just wasn't done in those days—maybe— at least not in our household.

Daddy's homebuilding days were often spent sitting on open houses. His homes were slow to sell and I think he grew tired of it. We always seemed to be living hand to mouth, even in such an upscale community as San Marino. Daddy worked part time for a San Marino realty company, answering phones and visiting with the realtors, until Mother got tired of worrying about money. In the want ads, she found a job for Daddy with the Los Angeles County Assessor's Office in downtown Los Angeles. He worked there for seven years and loved it, because he was around people all day in the office, and meeting more in their homes while doing assessing. Mother was happy again, and he retired with a pension and Social Security.

In 1957, it was time for their oldest child to start college; there was never an option whether we would go to college or not. Eileen took off for the University of San Diego and, luckily, Mother had a bachelor brother, Jimmy Anderson, who made quite a bit of money in the stock market, and he underwrote the first three Faherty college educations. We all were able to go away to private Catholic colleges, thanks to Uncle Jimmy, and then an aunt who took over when Jimmy died. I graduated from College of the Holy Names in Oakland, but Daddy was extremely happy when Santa Clara University became coed and Mary Ann was admitted to the second class that accepted women. Tom and Sheila also went there, although Joanie went to another Jesuit school, Seattle University. We didn't know who to thank until we graduated.

Things I remember about Daddy were: his wonderful sense of humor; his talent for drawing (we've had several of his pictures framed); taking Mother on tandem bicycle rides after dinner; attending daily Mass; kneeling down to say his prayers every night before going to bed; always saying grace before meals; writing us "Dear Brats," letters when away at college, often expounding upon who attended the funerals of friends and neighbors; playing bridge with friends, and with Dave and me after we were married, and hosting the annual St. Patrick's Day parties. I also remember when I told him (before we were married) that I was in love with David Recupero, his response was, "Isn't it just as easy to fall in love with a rich Irishman than a poor Italian?"; hating to go to the beach because he detested getting sunburned and sandy (the first time our son Michael heard Papa say "damn" was when Daddy was removing tar from his feet in our back yard); never tipping at restaurants, which embarrassed Mother terribly; being an impatient driver until Mother finally took the keys away when he was in his 70's; his competitiveness (he thrived on winning); falling back into his Southern accent when talking with others from the South; his prejudice against blacks, which he eventually overcame when one of his best friends at the County was a black woman (when we were young, if Nat King Cole or Ella Fitzgerald came on the TV, he would without a word go up and change the channel); vacationing with the family in Yosemite and Ojai (at a friend's ranch); his loyalty to his family, friends, the Catholic Church, Santa Clara, the Republican Party, and any Irishman. Our friends loved coming over to our house because he always welcomed everyone with the same, "Well, greetings."

Just six months after discovering he had cancer, Daddy died on April 23, 1987, of metastasized melanoma.

All who knew Daddy, know that he went on, with: "Well, greetings."

New York! New York! It's a Wonderful Town

Visiting New York is always exciting, but staying in Manhattan, which has a unique energy, is special. Dave and I had arrived on a Thursday with two other couples, for a five-day stay to see four plays. We had reserved rooms at the Warwick Hotel, which is in upper-midtown, about four blocks south of Central Park—a perfect location.

THE ERRANT ALARM CLOCK

It was the kind of alarm that gave off an annoying atonal ring, and on our first morning I was awakened by it in the next room. Lucky for Dave, he is hard of hearing (only "slightly," says he) because it didn't awaken him. I looked at our clock, four a.m., and thought, it will quit after a few minutes. It didn't quit . . . it didn't quit . . . and it didn't quit. I pressed zero on our phone to get the front desk. "The room seems to be empty next door and the alarm is going off and keeping me awake. Can you please have it turned off?"

"I will call security." a male voice said. Ten long minutes later, I heard a knocking on the door next to ours, the security guard letting himself in, and then the alarm went silent. Whew! I went back to sleep . . . eventually.

The next morning, again at four a.m., the same alarm went off, jolting me awake. This time I called the front desk immediately. Again, they sent up security to turn it off, and I was able to get back to sleep. When I eventually woke up that morning, and was coherent, I studied our alarm clock to see how it worked, but it was rather confusing. It turned out that you have to press two buttons simultaneously to turn off the alarm completely. If you press only one, it worked as a snooze alarm and reset the alarm to go off again at the same time—every day. Aha!

About four o'clock that afternoon, I heard someone unlock the door to the next room, probably someone moving in. To be a good neighbor I thought I would go and alert the new guests so they would not be disturbed by an errant alarm clock. Dave had hopped into the shower—we were dressing to meet our friends for cocktails before dinner and a play—so I didn't mention my leaving to him.

I knocked on the door next to ours. A woman opening the door about two inches, peeked out and said, "Yes?"

I explained to her, "The alarm in this room has gone off the prior two mornings at 4 a.m., waking me up. It's kind of a tricky alarm, so I wondered if you would mind if I came in and showed you."

She looked at me like I was some kind of a nutcase, one that possibly wanted to get in her room and do who knows what. She said, "No, I think I can take care of it."

I said, "But you have to push two . . ." The door closed, click—the dead bolt turned, clack. Well! I turned to go back into my room and realized that I hadn't brought my key; our door had automatically locked behind me, Dave was in the shower and couldn't hear me. I realized if I started knocking loudly to get his attention, the neighbor might think I was knocking on her door again, or that I was going room to room, all the while wondering if I needed some psychiatric help. Then it dawned on me: *She's right, I'm a nutcase.*

Well, it seemed she did know about alarm clocks—the alarm didn't go off the next morning, or I was so exhausted I slept right through it.

BREAKFAST AT RUE 57

We had tickets to see the Sunday two p.m., Tony Award winning show "Avenue Q." Never quite adjusting to New York time, we slept in late. Around noon, we decided to go for breakfast at Rue 57, a nice neighborhood French bistro-type restaurant about three blocks away, where we had eaten the previous morning. We soon found that Sunday brunch in Manhattan was a big deal, even when the temperature was hovering around 30 degrees in a nonresidential neighborhood on a nonbusiness day. So different from when we recently stayed over on a Saturday night in downtown Los Angeles, seeing *Doubt* at the Ahmanson theater and couldn't find an open restaurant on Sunday morning to walk to from the Omni Hotel, located only two blocks from the theater. Consequently, we ate at the hotel restaurant, which was good, but expensive.

At this Manhattan eatery, we inched our way into the front door to give our name to the maître d', then joined 20 other patrons who wanted tables. We observed at least two couples turn and walk out choosing not to wait. Everyone arrived in big coats, parkas, jackets, scarves, gloves, and hats. The tables were rather small and crowded in the large room, so there was a coat girl, probably in her mid-20's, begging everyone to check their coats. She herself was wearing a sexy strapped black camisole resembling a French burlesque dancer. It made one cold to look at her. Well, it made me cold; I don't know about Dave or the other elderly gentleman focused on her abundant cleavage.

The dark wood on the walls, 12-foot high ceilings, massive old, dark-wood bar with antique mirrors and brass trimmings, made the restaurant look like it had been in the neighborhood for over a century. Large orange glass and brass sconces provided warm lighting, and ten-foot palms in giant planters added a mellow green touch. As we stood waiting in the foyer, every time the door opened, an arctic draft reminded us of the outside cold, which was about every 45 seconds. The sign on the wall read, CAPACITY: 219 and there must have been at least that many people inside, not including the staff. Everyone was talking loudly to overcome the pounding music, but no one was paying attention to the upper corner over the bar where a TV was showing the latest bowling tournament. Bowling? How incongruous.

We were fortunate to find a seat in the foyer while waiting for our table, which gave us an excellent vantage point to observe the interesting aspects of managing a popular restaurant and its hungry crowd. We noticed that advance reservations were not an option but if you were friends of the maître d', he would slip you in within ten minutes instead of having to wait the regular 30 minutes. When we were finally seated, I asked the server if it was possible for us to be out the door in 45 minutes as we had tickets for a play. She said there would be no problem, and we believed her—after all, we just wanted scrambled eggs, toast and hot coffee.

Our coffee and French bread were delivered immediately, so we felt safe. Meanwhile the party next to us—and I mean next to us, a mere 18 inches away, left, and a young busboy came to clean and reset the table. After clearing the table, he returned with four glasses, four small plates, silverware for four and four linen napkins, all in his left hand. With his right hand he unfolded and spread out a white tablecloth, making it perfectly even and set the table—in less than 20 seconds: It was an artful performance.

Then they arrived: four New York matrons, well into their seventies. They didn't trust the coat girl with their paraphernalia, so they squeezed in next to us, bumping our table, carrying bulky full-length coats, scarves and gloves. One of the sleeves soaked up some of my coffee, but I figured she deserved it. After much loud discussion, they arrived at their menu decisions, two of them asked for, "Sliders with *pommes frites*." Sliders are small hamburgers about the size of a yoyo and come three to an order. The old woman with the coffee stained sleeve, ordered her sliders medium rare—emphatically, and loud enough for adjoining tables to hear.

Our orders arrived with only about 20 minutes to spare, so we didn't waste any time. Our eggs were perfectly cooked, the bread was toasted and delicious, similar to San Francisco sourdough, and the coffee was good, hot and plentiful. In addition, the persnickety matrons were entertaining.

When the women next to us received their meals, their questions started. The waiter was asked, "Is this medium rare?"

"Yes, Ma'am."

The waiter realized a mistake, and promptly brought wet-sleeve another plate. She asked again, "Is this medium rare?"

"Yes, Ma'am," he said.

"How do I know if you are telling me the truth? . . . You say yes to everything."

"It is medium rare, Ma'am."

"Humph!"

So why did we enjoy this busy, loud, crowded restaurant, and its long wait?

Because, it was soooooo New York.

Our Year in Tuscany

In June 2004, my husband Dave, and I decided to retire, hand over our consulting business to our son, and take off—to live in Italy for a year. One of our best friends, Chris Hickey, had recently died of prostate cancer and, being our same age of 63, his death reminded us that we never know what lies ahead for each of us.

We both loved to travel, had been to Italy a couple of times and, most importantly, Dave could speak a bit of Italian. I went on the Internet, read books, and studied maps for the perfect place to rent for a year. We wanted a home base from which to travel and see as much as we could of Europe. We decided on central Italy near the west coast, and chose Lucca, in Tuscany, between Pisa, and Florence. More a village than a big city, it had temperate weather, was within walking distance to the Lucca train station, and a 20-minute drive to the Pisa airport from which we could easily get around Europe. Our children, their spouses, and grandchildren would be able to visit for a couple weeks to observe Christmas, and so would many friends, especially those coming to attend the December 29 wedding of our daughter Sarah to Steve Ramos. Looking back, Dave and I both say that year was one of the best things we have ever done. Here are some vignettes of that special time and lovely place.

Lucca

Lucca is famous for being perhaps the largest Italian city with its medieval city wall still entirely intact, and for being the birthplace of opera great, Giacomo Puccini. Lucca's thick renaissance walls, medieval street plan, palaces and houses, and especially lack of tourists, give Lucca an exotic and foreign aura, which we found very exciting.

September 2004: Checking-in

Our first Italian "experience" upon arriving in Lucca was a misunderstanding concerning the apartment that we had booked online with Nicola and his agency. It turned out he doesn't speak or read English; he had Teà, a young student from Albania translating for him. Consequently, we got a two-bedroom instead of a three-bedroom, and learned that utilities were not included in the price agreed upon in his email.

We hammered out an agreement in his office. He would pay two of the three utilities, and in October, we could have the three-bedroom unit upstairs—for an increase of 200 Euros ($250) per month for the rest of the year.

In the two-bedroom apartment, we had a fairly new *matrimonial* bed (I think you have to be married to get one of these beds in Italy) that is similar to a queen size bed. The mattress was fine and all linens were provided. This apartment would do until October.

Montecatini, Our Mud Bath Experience

Shortly after settling in, we got brave and took our first excursion, two nights to Montecatini Terme, which is rated the top spa and resort in Tuscany. We were ready for some exploring and a pampering massage treatment. Upon my sister Mary Ann's recommendation, we stayed at the Hotel Suisse, and found the location perfect. Its large king size bed and huge new bathroom with Jacuzzi tub, were decadent treats. We enjoyed the ride on the 100-year old funicular railway up the side of a mountain to Montecatini Alto, with its grand view of the medieval town.

The next morning (at Dave's urging), just across the street, we signed up for a half-day, afternoon session at the famous spa, which included a mud treatment and massage. Never having had a mud bath (not even in Calistoga) I was reluctant, but Dave said we had to try everything—once. We arrived at our scheduled time of 14:00 (two p.m.) and were directed to the dressing rooms. The host asked us if we brought our own bathing suits. Yes, we replied—I was happy to learn that it was not nude bathing. We were shown to a room with a sauna, a steam room, a small shallow pool with cold water for walking around in, to soothe our feet I guessed, and some lounge chairs. Well, I hate to sweat—Dave loves to sweat. So I tolerated the first "relaxing hour" waiting for the massage hour to start. Eventually, we were called in for the mud treatment, and were put in adjacent rooms. A masseuse, a middle-aged woman, would do both of us. I was told to remove my robe and bathing suit, and was handed a cellophane package about as big as a package of Dentyne gum. I opened it to find a Kleenex-sized cover with two rubber bands attached, so I had a thong, and learned later that Dave got a windsock. I lay naked, waiting for the masseuse to finish with Dave, all the while listening to Indian music, alternating with Gregorian Chant. I couldn't help but laugh at myself and alternately cursing Dave. The masseuse finally came into my room and had me lay on a table covered with plastic. She soaped me on one side, had me turn over (I about slid off the table) and then soaped my other side. I then climbed into a huge Jacuzzi tub, and she turned on its scouring jets, roaring full speed ahead. Someone smaller than me would have had to do the backstroke to keep from washing away. She had me stay there for at least 45 minutes, while she tended to Dave.

I was prune-like when she allowed me to get out. She slobbered mud all over the back of me, and then had me lay on my back on a plastic sheet, while she mudded up my front side. Then she wrapped me in the plastic, like a mummy, so that I would sweat some more—I'm ready to clobber Dave. I was unable to move a muscle for about 30 minutes. I am not claustrophobic that I know of, but all of a sudden, understood the feeling. After a 15-minute shower to remove the inch of mud, and another Jacuzzi-jet pounding, I'm finally ready for the massage I've been craving for over the past two-hours. However, she tells me the massage starts at 17:00—my god, that's another 40 minutes. So I wait. She comes in, tells me Dave is sleeping, puts me on my stomach—yeah, finally—my massage. She puts cream on my back, does a 15-minute rubdown. Then says, "*Arrivederci!*" I say, "*Prego!*"

Dave and I meet in the lobby, and barely make it outside before we burst into laughter, agreeing that we've added another Italian *experience* to our growing list.

Moving Up in the World

October soon rolled around, and it was time to move upstairs into the three-bedroom apartment, and what an adventure it was. Because the tenant in the three-bedroom apartment above us was leaving, we asked him if he would leave the door unlocked so we could take a peek to see what supplies we were going to inherit, and if we needed to sneak anything of value from our current unit. While snooping around, waiting for the housekeeper so we could move in, the owner Paola entered. She was very gracious and glad to meet us—however, she spoke no English, so we did a lot of pointing—especially to the queen size bed set, with droopy, squeaky springs—that she expected us to sleep on for the next eleven months. We explained to her that we would like to change beds, to bring up our current queen size bed. After some hemming and hawing, she finally agreed—if we would do the work. *"Non problemo,"* said us confident Americans.

We soon found that we couldn't bring the upstairs bed-set down because it wouldn't fit into the stairwell. That's when I had the bright idea to lower it over the balcony. By this time, Tea, and her mother, Juliana (in her 70's), who was the woman in charge of cleaning the units, arrived and offered to help. Teà and I, on the third floor patio, lifted the spring set over the banister to lower it down to Dave and Juliana on the next balcony. We lowered it, with one white-knuckled hand each, as far as we could, but Dave and Juliana couldn't quite reach high enough. Now what! The bed-set was too heavy for us to lift back up—but then, my hero, Dave did the old high school stretch, and eased it into the second story patio. Job accomplished! Again, we had the nice, quiet, firm bed we had become used to, even though it was a little narrow for a couple used to an Eastern King size—we managed. Knowing we had logged another interesting Italiano esperienza.

CORTONA

Frances Mayes popularized Cortona in her best selling book, *Under the Tuscan Sun,* a reason we decided to take a sojourn there for a couple of days. While we were packing, Dave asked me if he should pack any *dress-up* clothes, and I told him we were only going to be hiking through a couple of hill towns, so just jeans and a couple of clean shirts should be fine.

On our way, we decided to make a dry run to see if we could find the *Firenze* (Florence) train station where we would be picking up family and friends. Unfortunately, unlike the Orange County Airport, right off the freeway, the *Firenze* train station is in *Centro,* about 10–15 minutes off the *Autostrada.* We found it okay, with only one wrong turn, but finding our way back to the *Autostrada* to continue our trip to Cortona was a challenge. The direction signs in most of the larger cities in Europe usually take a minimum of two people, first to find the sign, and then to understand it. We found ourselves going in circles, with me commenting, "Look, Dave, there's the duomo (cathedral); look, Dave, there's the duomo; look, Dave . . ."

Cortona is about an hour and a half from Florence, and during the drive, I researched my various travel books and found a charming place where I wanted to stay. *Il Falconiere* was listed in Karen Brown's *Italy* (if you've never heard of *karenbrown.com* you may want to look at her website). Since it was a Tuesday, I didn't call to make reservations and thought we'd do a "drive-by" first. The place was listed as "on the road to Cortona." Well, we made it to Cortona without ever seeing the place, and now it was getting dark. All we could see were olive trees, vineyards, more olive trees, a corn field, a church (of course), and on a dead-end street, a small *cemetario* with the obligatory statue of Mary adorned with enough flowers to open a nursery. I pleaded with Dave to make another run at it, and managed to see a tiny sign for *Il Falconiere,* on the side of the road. After what seemed like miles on wavy dirt roads in the dark, we arrived at what was quite an estate. Il Falconiere had a vacancy, and would we like to join them for dinner? Would we like some wine while waiting for the 20:00 dinner? Now we were cruisin'.

I was a little nervous about dinner. Il Falconiere was more upscale than I had planned. I had only my new black Italian jeans (sleek with no pockets, but with orange stitching—darn!), a black sweater, but had not brought jewelry. Dave cheated, and brought nice pants and a sweater. I thought, what the heck, we're not going to see anyone we know. Well, at the table, on our right was a couple from Australia—she with her fur-collared sweater set, long skirt, and dripping with jewelry. It turned out they own a home and vineyard in Montecatini Alta where they reside six months out of the year, and live the other six months in Australia. All that went through my mind was: Did she notice the orange stitching? Was it so dim in the dining room that she thought I was dressed appropriately in black wool? On the other side of us sat a couple from Poland, both *dressed for dinner*. For years a mathematics professor, he had started his own computer company in Poland, twelve years ago. She was translating the Encyclopedia Britannica into Polish from English—not your average nine-to-five job. People loved to talk with us when they heard English spoken. Next time, I am bringing jewelry and dressy pants.

Early the next morning, Dave went out to pick olives with the field crew, they sang Italian folk songs while picking. Il Falconiere makes its own olive oil and its own wine. In the afternoon, Silvia, the owner-wife, gave us a tour of their olive oil factory, and that evening, Ricardo, the owner-husband gave us a tour of their estate and winery. There was one other California couple staying there that took the estate tour—she was an attorney from Hermosa Beach, and he was a CPA from Murrieta. We soon became friendly, and on the second night, had dinner together—orange stitching again. When checking out, the owner told us that if we stayed another night we would meet Ms. Frances Mayes, a good friend of theirs, who would be eating dinner there, celebrating her newly published book, *Bringing Home Tuscany*. But my jeans were wrinkled, and I had to go home.

FLU SHOTS

It was wintertime so we decided to get flu shots, so we would not get sick at Christmas time, with family and friends scheduled for the holiday, and the upcoming wedding. There was no shortage of vaccine in Italy, as we had heard there was in the U.S. We asked Norma Bishop, an American who has a 24 hour help service called "A Friend in Tuscany," She had lived twelve years in France and this was her ninth year in Lucca. Norma took us to her *dottore,* who starts her office hours in the afternoon, at 15:00. There were about seven people before us, so we waited in line on stairs in a hallway—no appointments, with first come, first served. When our turn finally came, Dr. Banducci ushered us into her office, questioned why we were there, and promptly wrote us a prescription. She then instructed us to take it to a pharmacy. The pharmacy sold us a syringe and the vaccine for seven and a half Euros (nine dollars). We then went back to the doctor's office and stood in line again. She gave us the shot, but was not allowed to take any money, even though we offered and told her we were visitors. My kind of medical system.

THANKSGIVING

Many have asked if we celebrated Thanksgiving while in Lucca. We certainly did. About two weeks before Thanksgiving and after searching quite a few *mercati,* we found a poultry-shop where we could order a *whole* turkey—unheard of in Italy. I asked the butcher for about a 15-pounder, but they, of course, go by kilograms. He didn't understand, so I showed him how big with my hands. The butcher asked us how many people we were having for dinner. I said nine—he burst out laughing, in fact doubled over—I was sure he thought we were feeding about fifty.

After ordering the turkey, it took us a week to find a shop that carried a meat thermometer. When I tried to explain to the shopkeepers what I wanted, they understood the thermometer part, but they only sell them for taking the temperature of people. When I said *per carne o pollo* they gave me a weird look, like I was kinky or something. Finally, Dave found one made in Germany that, of course, was in Celsius. Not a worry, with my math major background, I translated to Fahrenheit.

When I picked up the turkey on the Wednesday before Thanksgiving, you would not believe the reception I got from other women in the shop. One old lady asked the butcher what it was when she saw him bring the turkey out of the locker. She had never seen a whole turkey, and there was a lot of excited chatter in the shop. A young gal in the shop then asked me if I was American and if we were celebrating Thanksgiving. She had seen it in the movies. Thank God the head feet and feathers were removed, and the inside cleaned out— and I mean cleaned out—no giblets, neck, or organs.

We had nine people for dinner, with a mother and her son (age five) from Arkansas, a grandmother with her daughter and son (age five) from Norway; and niece Katy and her friend Callie, both studying in *Firenze*. Both girls grew up together in Woodland, CA. The Norwegians had never had turkey dressing, cranberry sauce, or a salad with candied walnuts, feta cheese and pears. They loved this new food, and appreciated the invitation to dinner. Siri said she had heard of Thanksgiving, and now wanted to take the custom back with her to Norway. In the afternoon, while I prepared the dinner, Dave got all kinds of things ready for the five-year olds to play with. He had them hunting for presents, making turkeys out of oak leaves, and forming words out of homemade letter tiles. Only when they were leaving did we learn that the Norwegian five-year old was the only one in the group who didn't speak or understand English. His mother and grandmother did so well, we had assumed that he understood us also. He smiled so much I was sure he picked up something that night. It was such a fun evening that we almost didn't miss our traditional, annual, family Thanksgiving celebration at my brother's home in the Napa Valley. And, thank goodness, there was more celebration ahead, with lots of relatives and friends, coming to Medieval Lucca for the holiday and the wedding.

A POSTCARD FROM LUCCA

All the waiting and counting down worked, Christmas and the wedding are over, and here in Lucca, at one in the morning, I'm sitting at my computer, with tears in my eyes. Our children and friends have left for home, and I'm asking myself, did I hug Annie hard enough and tell her how much I appreciated all her hard work? Did I kiss the grandsons enough for they will be inches taller when I see them again? Did I tell Johnny H. how much I love his quiet presence and patience with the boys? Did I take enough time with our son Mike and Lauren, because the next time I see them they will be new parents? But, still; daughter Sarah and Steve arrive back from their honeymoon in Cinque Terre tomorrow morning, for a short visit before leaving for home on Tuesday.

What a fabulous time we had! Christmas was never better with 24 of us sitting down to dinner (albeit "kids" on the stairs—anyone 21 and under). After dinner, we enjoyed a couple of hours of Texas Hold'em with packages of Splenda used as poker chips. Anne and Lauren showed up the guys by coming away winners. There was lots of laughter, and the noise level was high: music to our ears.

And then on December 29th, the WEDDING! A once-in-a-lifetime event. It truly was a fairy tale wedding, held in beautiful *chiesa* San Pietro Somaldi built in 1199, and the dinner reception in a palace, Palazzo Pfanner, once owned by the Duke of Lucca. The palace, built in the 1600s, had murals on the ceiling and walls. Sarah got her wish to be able to walk through the ancient cobblestone streets in her white dress and veil, to the church—no rain. The 30-member procession that followed them included a wonderful French priest from Limoges, a cousin of son-in-law John, who came by train to Lucca to witness the wedding and say the Mass for Steve and Sarah. (Only later did we learn that it took him 24 hours to get from France to Italy because of his remote location in the Pyrenees.) Grandsons Matt & Will were altar boys. The music performed by a string quartet and an Italian vocalist brought tears to our eyes. The seven-course Tuscan banquet served by waiters wearing white gloves, was indescribably delicious. We even had some Italian friends attend, including an AFS student we hosted in 1987, who now lives in Genoa. What a treat to see him again, and husband Dave was very taken by Gabriella, his gorgeous fiancée.

So why do I have tears in my eyes when everything was perfect? Because everything was perfect and it's all over.

BACK TO EVERYDAY LIFE IN LUCCA

It was January, and the average temperature was in the low 30's, when our tank-less water heater went kaput. The electrical *reset button* was not resetting, so no hot water and, because our apartment was warmed by the same system, no heat. Upon calling our property manager, she said she would call a plumber and he would be out that afternoon. He didn't show. Now we had been living there almost five months, and we were reluctantly getting used to the Italian way of life, but I must add, thoroughly enjoying it also. So we waited, and called the following afternoon to see if he was coming. She didn't know nor did she seem worried about it, because after all, she "had left a message for him." Since she didn't seem to appreciate the seriousness of the situation, Dave told the agent that the rent would be withheld as long as it took to get a plumber. A plumber was at our door in 20 minutes! Amazing how you can eventually pick up on the Italian culture. We found out later that workers were not allowed to drive their trucks within the walls that surrounded the city. If they had a job inside, it meant parking in one of six parking lots on the periphery of the town, paying for parking, and then walking with their heavy tools, perhaps a mile to the job. So unless it was worth their time and effort, they just didn't show up. Only homeowners with special stickers could drive and park within the walls.

Lent in Lucca

The doorbell sounded one day, and that being a very rare occasion, I looked out the window to see who it might be before buzzing the door open. I saw a rather elderly monsignor standing on our doorstep (I assumed he was a monsignor because he was wearing a purple hat and stole). I called out a *buon giorno* and rang him in. Huffing and puffing, he managed to climb the three flights of stairs. I suspected he arrived to bless our house because it was Ash Wednesday, and he was carrying a holy water sprinkler and a small prayer book. He didn't speak English, but I understood his one word: *Cattolica?* I answered *si, si,* and he proceeded to sprinkle some holy water around and said some prayers either in Italian or Latin, I wasn't sure. I also wasn't sure if he was doing an exorcism, or if this was a Lenten tradition. I hoped for the latter. Afterwards, I did feel a bit easier about living there—maybe we would continue to have hot water, electricity, and phone service until we checked out.

ORVIETO

We made another excursion, this time to Orvieto, a hill town in Umbria, a short distance north of Rome. Besides its ceramics, and the exquisite *duomo* (cathedral), Orvieto is famous for its labyrinth of Etruscan caves dug right under the city. We toured the caves, climbing down about three stories, and learned that during the Second World War, the locals used the caves as a bomb shelter. It is said that if Orvieto had been bombed, the city might have collapsed right into the caves. I was a little nervous, praying there would not be an earthquake while we were under a city of 10,000 people.

We thoroughly enjoyed our two-night stay at the *agriturismo* (farm) Locanda Rosati. Located in the valley below Orvieto, Locanda Rosati was owned and run by Giampiero and his brother-in-law Paolo. They both mingled with their guests, answered questions, and suggested things for us to do, and hosted a family style dinner every night, which most of the guests attended. We ate there both nights, enjoying the company of travelers from Saudi Arabia, Italy, Canada, Chicago, and San Francisco. From Saudi Arabia were two British women who worked for a Saudi oil company because they could make much more money than in England. They lived in a self-contained compound and rarely left it because of the danger, so for them, it was a big treat to be in Italy. Everyone had interesting stories to tell. The dinner, spiced with interesting conversation, lasted over three hours.

Before dinner, Giampiero had to drive out to his cousin's dairy farm to pick up some fresh milk for that night, and asked Dave and I if we wanted to accompany him. Well, what a great opportunity. At the *agriturismo,* I thought we were already in the country, but after driving about five kilometers we arrived at a tiny village (population 150), it was *really* in the country. We traversed three switchbacks to get to his cousin's barn, where there were 50 cows, a few bulls, and one ten-day old calf. Giampiero took a hose connected to a machine and filled his bottle with milk. I didn't ask if it was pasteurized, homogenized, or whatever, but it was indeed fresh.

CHIANTI REGION

The week after Easter we picked up some old college friends in Florence and drove down to some of the hill towns southwest of Siena: Montepulciano, Pienza, and Montalcino. I think this is my favorite scenery in all of Italy. It is truly postcard picturesque, rolling hills, cypress trees, and villas on hilltops. We stayed amid the hills in a lovely small hotel, with a beautiful view of Pienza (population: 2200), and its magnificent duomo and papal palace. Pienza has one main street "Piazza Pio II" with upscale shops, one of which had a wonderful pungent Pecorino cheese wrapped in black wax, and an exquisite Brunello wine. We thoroughly enjoyed eating at the *Trattoria Latte di Luna* (milk of the moon); even the *Wall Street Journal* wrote about it.

One afternoon, after a few wrong turns, we finally found the Abbey Sant'Antimo, which I had read about and wanted to hear Benedictine monks chant their prayers in Latin. For twenty enchanting minutes, it seemed like we were back in medieval times—that is, until the monks hopped into their small Fiat and tore down the dusty road with their white robes flying. That sort of ruined the experience. I hoped they weren't going for an American experience of burgers and fries at a McDonalds.

Saying Goodbye to a Wonderful Year

Reluctant to leave, we were nevertheless ready to go home. We had taken the last of our packed boxes to Mailbox Etc. to be shipped home to California. We had said our goodbyes to Beppe, the wedding florist, who always gave me free flowers when I poked my head in to say *ciao;* Ciro the deli man, the first Lucchese we spoke with when we arrived, starved, and wide eyed; Nicola and Cristina, our agents, who by the way gave us our deposit back the morning before we left (does this happen in the States?); Jennifer, the girl from New Jersey who came to Lucca to study Italian and ended up marrying a sweet Italian man, Paolo (we ended up giving them many of our Italian furnishings which we couldn't take back to the States); Angela, the maître d' who called out "*Signora Recupero*" when we entered our favorite restaurant last night, double kissed us, and almost cried when we said we had to go home on *Mercoledi;* Stefano, whom I've fallen in love with, even if he can't speak English—I could tell in his eyes that he's in love with me (but he's too young)—any time you are in Lucca, be sure and eat at Al Porto, his restaurant; the lady next door who exclaimed *"Bravo, bravo"* when I gave her my cashmere wool coat which I bought for 13-Euros at a street market, and who sewed up Dave's pajamas when he split the seam (we joined Weight Watchers when we got home); Norma, who wrapped up our account with Telecom and thankfully disconnected us in a shorter period of time than the weeks it took to connect us; Michel and Gina, our French-American friends who helped us at the Internet Café way back in the Fall.

We drove our car to *Pisa Aeroporto,* dropped it off, and then boarding our flight said *arrividerci* to a wonderful year, a year that flew by far too fast, yet gave us treasured memories to hold on to for the rest of our lives.

William (Bill) Reid

Among the hundreds of senior citizens with whom I've worked, none has been more successful at recapturing an era and the author's place in that era than Bill Reid. One thinks inevitably of the pit towns in Sons and Lovers or the landscapes in Return of the Native, or of Angela's Ashes. It seems to me that writings such as Bill Reid's memoirs are infinitely valuable, being, as it were, "the real thing," lived history.

When Bill first entered the workshop, he was writing a "thriller," The Aztec Princess. I like to think that some of my reactions and suggestions and those of other participants helped him refine this tale. When he switched to the stories from his personal history, we had little to say, except that we found his work fascinating and moving. No doubt, my enthusiasm for the memoirs and my tepid interest in the thriller reflect my own reading tastes. I just don't like thrillers, and I do much enjoy personal narrative—Roughing It and Life on the Mississippi, for example.

—W.R.W.

There's a War On!

For the British Isles, World War II started on September 3, 1939. Anticipating German air raids, the British government imposed an immediate nationwide blackout, and issued gas masks to everyone, including tots and babies. On January 8, 1940, the government instituted rationing of food and many other essential items. Six days later, I celebrated my tenth birthday in Lochgelly, a small coal-mining town in the Shire of Fife, Scotland—the peninsula just North of Edinburgh, whose map is a profile of a Scottie dog.

All but the first two years of my life had been spent in shared-living arrangements, usually the use of a bedroom in homes rented by others. My father, as a deep-pit coal miner, like his father and brother, was often unemployed because of lack of work or because of work-related accidents. Dad could not afford to rent even a tenement home. As the war in Europe was developing, coalminers found full-time employment, and Dad was able to get a home for us in the *Happyland*. The Happyland, so named by the town council, was a complex of soot-stained brick, two-story, rowhouse tenements, constructed for coal miners. Built on the eastern edge of town, the complex covered what had once been the town common, where gypsies camped and farmers offered goods and services for sale. The Happyland was an overt project to oust one of the three major, reviled and feared gypsy bands in Scotland. Our two-room, lower level house, facing East, had a view of pastoral farmland and distant woods, that was negated by the Jenny Gray pug, a steam locomotive (a Thomas the Tank Engine) that, frequently, on the other side of a wall only 20 yards from our home, hauled eight carloads of freshly mined coal from the adjacent Jenny

Gray coal mine, to an incline system that would lower the cars to the Nellie pit, for washing—separating from shale, and screening by size. We tried to ignore the pug's noisy clatter, and its steam-belched billows of sooty, sulphur-smelling smoke that smudged our clothing and tainted our existence.

In the early weeks of the war, our parents' anxiety was made worse by the frenetic and sometimes confusing actions of the government. However, happily settled into our wee Happyland home some months earlier, I found, like other school kids had, that I was far more interested in real-time happenings, than the disruptions, restrictions, and rumors that had our parents distracted and fussing. To us kids, war was just another interest, and to better enjoy the war, we kept up with the news. To us, war was exciting stuff!

Our main news source, the British Broadcasting Company (BBC), had an evening news broadcast that always started with updates on the war effort, followed by details on the latest war-mandated regulatory changes. I huddled every evening with Dad, Mum, and my sister, Jessie, listening to the news warbling from the tinny speaker in our Marconi radio receiver. If our only accumulator (battery) faded, we missed important news. My chore before school on Fridays was to lug the heavy lead-acid radio battery, changing hands every twenty or so steps, to a shed three blocks away that was attached to the back of a home owned by a grizzly-bearded old man. He re-charged batteries for friends, although his home was not a licensed business. The weirdly throbbing hum from the Frankenstein-like equipment and tangled wiring that seemed to reach for me, at times made more frightening by the shuddering rumble of the Jenny Grey pit pug clattered by next to the shed. I always quickly set the battery on the floor at the door of his shed and scooted home, the short way, along the pug-tracks to the wall near our home.

Dad always picked up the charged battery on his way home from work, and put the battery in the radio for the Friday evening news. A particular piece of stirring drum-music always heralded the BBC evening news. As an aspiring drummer, I often drummed along with my fingertips, sometimes on the shoulders of my younger sister. Two years apart, Jessie and I were very close. A sweet but timid soul, she never complained about anything. As the introductory music faded, a precise voice, devoid of emotion, droned the important news events: Hitler's onslaught of Poland; the Blitzkrieg of France; the evacuation of Dunkirk; the Battle of Britain; and then, the latest on the previous night's air raids—the blitz. Aged now, to a respectable 77 years, I retain clear memories of that time; and, too, of another radio voice—a confident voice, a dominant presence, a robust, resolute, reassuring voice—of a man upon whom my father, mother, and grandmother heaped derision, on his every broadcast. Winston Churchill had said, back in 1926, that machine guns should be used against striking coal miners. United under trade unions, mineworkers were a potent force—who knew well that the country survived in part on coal and the men who risked their lives to mine it. Despite Dad's anger at our prime minister, I liked listening to Winston Churchill; just like the drum music, he stirred me.

Along with the war came posters with slogans and cautionary sayings—morale building propaganda that seeped into our psyche:

> There's a War On!
> Careless Talk Costs Lives
> Dig For Victory
> Keep On Smiling
> Always Carry Your Gas Mask
> Keep it Under Your Hat
> Potatoes Make Good Soup
> Join The Women's Land Army
> V is For Victory
> Your Courage Will Bring Us Victory

"There's a war on!" became a common saying to emphasize the importance of essential matters, and to justify hardships imposed on people, including school children.

Air raid shelter construction had commenced, and the dangers of explosive and incendiary bombs were made plain to everyone. Speedy German light-bombers, we were told, would start an air raid by dropping incendiary bombs to create a blazing directional path and a circle of fire around industrial area targets. Flying high, heavy-bombers would follow the fiery path and drop high-explosive bombs within the ring of fire. Although on the path to many key targets, Lochgelly had more of a risk from incendiary devices than from explosive bombs.

Incendiary bombs were simple in design, but effective devices. They were just a magnesium case filled with nasty stuff and magnesium chips that, when ignited, gave a frightful roar as they sprayed sun-bright blue-white fire out one end for about ten minutes. Enough time to set a structure ablaze after crashing through a roof, its almost unquenchable blaze burning through ceilings and floors. Bomber pilots simply followed a trail of blazing structures to their main targets. We were also told that householders and willing children could control incendiaries—to save lives and homes—as a contribution to the war effort. At morale booster meetings, we were shown British incendiary bombs, which looked like an aluminum tube, about eighteen inches long and perhaps two inches in diameter. Military experts demonstrated how to control the hellish fire of incendiaries, using sandbags and stirrup pumps. Adults and willing youngsters were trained to control incendiary bombs, using one of two techniques, against a roaring, fire spitting, acrid smelling incendiary device. I was willing, and although only ten, I said, "I want to do Method Two. Me . . . Me . . ." waving my arms. But, like others my age, I live-drilled only on Method One.

Method One: The least scary, called for approaching the blazing incendiary from the side, carrying a sand-filled bag high on my chest, as a face shield, peeking over the bag as needed, to get close enough to dump the bag over the *angry* end of the incendiary—then to scamper back to get a pail of water and a stirrup pump. The sandbag was not to extinguish the incendiary, but stop the spread of fire. The stirrup pump, with Mum or Jessie fetching water, was to help me control any fire that might have been started by an incendiary. Scary, scary—I had volunteered—but had soon wanted out when I saw others do it. Shame is stronger than common sense. Even though the sandbag was heavy, and I was small for my age, I managed to dump a sandbag over the fire-spitting end, and squirted water at a nearby fire simulated by burning wood. I appreciated Dad's nod of approval.

Method Two: demonstrated by experts using British incendiary bombs, was to be used in the absence of sandbags, or an inability to get a sandbag onto the incendiary. Although a very scary procedure, Dad did well when he live-drilled. I watched others do it, carefully, because when Dad was at work, I was to be the team captain for our Happyland home. I did one practice on a burned-out incendiary, where carrying a pail of water with a stirrup pump ready in the pail, I approached the open end of the device, to about six to eight feet distant, and positioned at a 45-degree angle (so as to not be blinded or spattered by the incendiary), and with a foot on the base of the stirrup pump, I pumped with one arm while reaching out with the hose nozzle to direct a jet of water at the nasty end of the bomb—a very hit-or-miss proposition—because the pump only squirted water on the down-stroke. Mum or Jessie brought water to the pail that fed the pump. I continued till the bomb fizzled out, then, with the thumb-slide on the nozzle switched to spray mode, to control any fire it had started. I found out many years later, unlike the incendiaries we trained with, German incendiary bombs added phosphor, a material that made incendiaries almost impossible to extinguish. Phosphor can auto-ignite if exposed to air—the water (H_2O), sprayed at an incendiary, provided hydrogen and oxygen—causing German incendiaries to burn out sooner—as a way to reducing the spread of fire. The military did not confuse us with such facts.

Lochgelly schoolboys who underwent sandbag and stirrup pump training to control incendiary bombs, had serious bragging rights—so, too, did the few girls who *had-to-show* the boys. I learned later that the training of homeowners and kids had proven effective, because the government credited sandbags and stirrup pumps as having saved many homes in areas targeted with incendiaries. No incendiary bombs fell on Lochgelly, and only two explosive bombs hit our town. One killed a fat old sheep in a field outside of town, and the other, an unexploded bomb that narrowly missed our local gas-works, was safely defused by a brave team of experts. Shrapnel, from the exploded shells of our own ack-ack (anti-aircraft) guns, was a different matter. Although capable of killing a person in the open, shrapnel never penetrated our roofs, but only damaged roofing slates and broke a few windows. I never heard of any injuries, and, like other kids, collected shrapnel as war souvenirs—even sharpening pencils with the sometimes razor-edged pieces.

After the war, stirrup-pumps had another use—for spreading liquid fertilizer (a strained emulsion made with hand-gathered sheep-doo) on Dad's victory plot. I helped Dad grow vegetables: kale, brussels sprouts, cabbages, cauliflower, turnips, beets, carrots, onions, celery, parsley and mint—for soups and stews; rhubarb and gooseberries for jams and desserts.

The sandbags used for incendiary control were made from burlap filled with dry sand, measuring about a foot in diameter and two feet long. Extra bags, available at a very low cost from the local town council, served as ideal sacks for youngster to use while scrounging (gleaning) potatoes from recently harvested fields. A great budget extender and pantry filler for families in the Happyland housing tract, scrounging was an important weekend activity. Some farmers welcomed us for eliminating tubers that could sprout into their next crop. Others would chase us off their property; a few even sicced their dog at us. I spent many weekends scrounging whole and damaged potatoes from recently harvested fields; Jessie sometimes came with me. A full sandbag of potatoes was as much as I could carry on my shoulder; Jessie less than half a bag. At nearby fields we did two sessions in a day. Lochgelly sat on the crown of a hill, the highest point in Fife, so the walk home, at times a mile or so, was always uphill. Rain before a scrounging session exposed more potatoes, but inches of soil that stuck to the soles of our boots made the going heavy. Nevertheless, the effort and hardship of scrounging proved rewarding. We garnered a generous supply of wonderful potatoes to store in our dark coal shed.

We knew potatoes as *spuds,* but more often as *tatties,* pronounced *tawt'is,* and much like the Irish, potatoes were a major part of our diet and an integral part of our life, particularly during harvest season. A major crop throughout the extensive farming areas of Fife, potatoes provided seasonal employment for senior citizens, housewives, and others during the near-winter chill of late September and October. In 1939, World War II military conscription (compulsory draft) took all able-bodied men not employed in essential industries (the coal mines and farms, for example). Women who did not enlist in women's militia, took factory jobs, or joined the newly created Women's Land Army, thus releasing men from their essential employment category of farming, to enlist in the military services. My mother's youngest sister and her friend joined the Land Army. They worked together in central Fife doing regular farm work—but no potato picking! School kids had become an alternate work force for the potato harvest in the war years.

During WWII, many school children ten and older were recruited to work in the potato fields, including me. I started when ten years of age, in 1940. During the war, school holiday closures adapted to accommodate potato harvesting. Summer recess in Scotland, normally in June and July—changed to only three weeks in June, plus four or five weeks in late September and most of October—for the potato harvest. School kids were strongly encouraged to pick potatoes, but earned much less than the amount paid to adult harvesters. Fife is at Latitude 56 degrees North, whereas Bangor, Maine in the United States, for example, is only at the North Latitude of 49 degrees. Fife gets long summer days to grow bountiful potato crops, and the shorter fall days bring frosty nights. Potatoes have a better taste and texture when the top growth is shriveled by heavy frosts. The cold North Sea that washes the peninsula of Fife averages 48 degrees in September-October, so cold, misty, often-drizzly conditions prevail—perhaps the impetus that created the fieriness of Scottish whiskeys.

Fife schoolchildren who agreed or were coerced to pick potatoes, had to leave home before 6:00 am. When going to pick potatoes, I had to walk through a blacked-out town, usually frosty, with only a feeble, torch (flashlight), hooded to restrict the light beam downward, to get to the farmers' pickup station. If I were even a few minutes late in meeting a farmer who had me for the day, he might cuff my ear. Wearing a balaclava, a thick-wool whole head and neck garment, gave protection from more than just the icy chill.

In that era, schoolboys did not wear, or even own, long pants until they finished school at age fourteen. For potato picking, pant legs would have soon been soaked and caked to become unmanageable—bare legs worked best. Girls, picking tatties, too, wore skirts well above the knee, and pushed their socks down to their boots. We did, however, dress well from the waist up, with a thick underwear layer, a flannel shirt, a wool sweater (or even two), a thick jacket that reached to just below the waist; and sturdy leather boots.

In a drawstring cloth-bag, we carried cheese sandwiches that were wrapped in lots of torn sheets of newspaper. The newspaper had supplementary uses. Each of us carried our gas mask in its bulky rectangular box on a strap hung around our neck. We often suffered transits of an hour or more in the back of an open lorry (truck), jostled on rough roads with nothing more than a loose tarp to cover us, and sometimes only a folded tarp to sit on. I found some farmers to be mean spirited taskmasters (stingy callous bastards), who abused us kids, even though we were doing our best for the war effort. As I write, I remember those heartless farmers, yet I still have proud memories of my war-effort potato picking experiences.

I recall many mornings, chilled through, on a potato field soon after dawn, with a farmer assigning me a stint. A stint that was perhaps twelve yards or more long—depending on the length of the field and number of people picking—factors that set how often the tractor would come around and scatter a potato row. My strongest memory is my first morning, standing in a field of long furrows running between potato rows covered with frost-killed tops, shivering like the other boys and girls. My gloveless fingers, curled into claws by the numbing cold, are clutching a two-bushel wire basket. My bare knees are knocking as I watch a belching, blotchy-green monster approaching. It's an impressive mechanical creature, a design perhaps inspired by a tyrannosaurus, in that it has tiny front wheels bobbing up and down in the furrows while giant rear wheels power it forward. Roaring and spewing acrid fumes as it nears, the monster's whirling tail is scattering a potato row. A fiend sits on the monster's back, a fiend so well disguised in bulky clothing that only black eyes scowl through slits in a dark-red, full-head balaclava helmet. As the monster passes a marker stake, the start of my stint, I hustle behind it, drop onto my bare knees, and pushing the basket ahead of me, pick and scoop potatoes into the basket. As soon as the basket is full enough, I drag it some three yards to the side, snag another basket from a row of empties, and repeat the gathering process. Numerous baskets will have been filled and dragged aside by the time I reach the marker that starts the next potato picker's stint. There, I move that stint marker one furrow over, resisting the urge to fudge a few inches. By then, the blotchy-green monster will once again be roaring near, urged on by the fiend with a metronome for a heart.

With soil caked thick on boots and knees, I hobble back to the start of my stint. Standing aside, three yards away from the row smitten by the monster's paddles, stray dirt clods strike my bare legs as I cringe away from the passing fiend and the dangerous twirling tail of his menacing mount. The six red paddles of its tail are swatting the side of the furrow, swop–swop–swop, converting the raised-row from a flat-topped pyramid to a formless swath. After it passes, I step into my stint, arch my back to help straighten a stooped-over set, and peer along the length of my stint. I see that the whirling paddles have strewn the row and its rich hoard over a six-foot width of my stint. There are potatoes of all sizes, withered plant tops and stringy white roots, dirt clods and stones, and too, blood-red worms, obscenely fat—writhing in agitation at such a rude awakening. The freshly disturbed soil, steaming slightly in the chilly morning air, exudes a loamy earthiness; a nose with hints of sliced potatoes and ruptured worms, amid an overt overtone of cow-dung from the spring planting.

At my stint marker, I heave a resigned sigh, let the basket drop, and plop onto my knees—not to pray—to again remember what my dad had told me, "It's tough work, but you're a coal miner's son. You can work hard. You can put up with discomfort." Then, of course— "There's a war on!"

Ahead of me, I hear the fiend rein his monster to a stop—someone's in trouble—a kid no doubt. I shudder at the thought of what the fiend might do. Woe is the picker who has not cleared his stint when the fiend arrives to scatter the next row, because the fiend is empowered to swing his rubber-booted foot. On my numb knees, the wide swath of my picking stretch requires that I zigzag my way along the stint, to gather all the potatoes larger than about an inch, immature potatoes will fall through the basket mesh. I pick and I scoop, left hand and right hand, basket after basket, while groveling all the way to the distant marker; too mindful of the fiend's boot to remember that, "There's a war on."

The farmers (*Brutes,* to us kids) usually spent the first part of the morning assigning and adjusting stints such that no child got a rest after clearing a stint. They set the tractor speed based on experienced adults paid by the hour for an agreed on stint length. A few brutes started school kids with excessively long stints, berating, and even cuffing or booting a few as their brutal method to set a demanding pace. Even the farmers that set tolerable stints angered easily at any tractor delays.

At times, perhaps more brutal, was the weather. Fife, situated between the Firth of Forth to the south and the Firth of Tay to the north, is a peninsula in the cold North Sea. Soaking mists and light rains were never reason enough to stop picking. In wet conditions, the professional pickers wore oilskin jackets and pants over regular clothing. So too did Brute and his pet fiend. All us kids had home-knitted wool gloves—useless for picking potatoes—but valuable during chilly transits in the farmer's lorry. So we endured the throb of fingers bent to form claws.

Always miserable in the early hours of the first few days, we nevertheless coped, and adapted to bear the cold, and toughened to endure the demanding pace. We felt the reward of pride in our worthy accomplishments of doing grownups jobs in the face of bitter weather and insensitive treatment. We also appreciated the times when warm and sunny periods made the job easier. And, we always knew that when we got home from potato picking there would be a toasty coal fire, a hot water scrub, and a big bowl of tattie-leek, or split-pea soup, with toast. Then, bedtime, the warm embrace of a cozy feather mattress and a down quilt, and dreams of sunshine. I slept well on those nights, never noticing the warbling *Air Raid* siren wails, alerting us that a bombing raid was imminent, or later, the steady sonorous siren drone that signaled the *All Clear*.

I was thirteen (1943) when I rebelled against a particularly brutal farmer. I called him *Beast*. His farm, west of Lochgelly, even well west of Dunfermline (the ancient capital of Scotland), was in a location remote from villages and bus routes. Assigned with three friends, boys of my age (older boys usually went to the farthest farms), we found that we were the only kids on Beast's potato field. Beast set us excessive stints, ranted throughout the day, and at times inflicted pain with his hand, and occasionally swung a wellington (knee-length rubber boot) protected foot. Complaints made Beast angrier, and since no adults took our side, and we needed him for transportation home, we put up with his ranting and cuffing. In his farmyard at lunchtime, we were abused enough to try to even the score. Instead of snitching the usual potatoes, we filched six or so hen eggs from his barn roosts, wrapping the eggs in crumpled newspaper, and packing them in our gasmask box and sandwich bag. Half a dozen fresh eggs each was a big score—considering that the government ration was only one egg per-person per-week as a whole-food supplement to the tasteless powdered-egg substitute that completed our ration. That evening, it was near dark when Beast unloaded us in Lochgelly. All four of us immediately complained to the volunteer School Farm Help Coordinator (the Tattie Gaffer to us), an old age pensioner. The Gaffer told us that Beast was new on his roster, and he would sort things out with him in the morning. Then, with his promise to tame Beast, he talked us into going back to Beast's farm—his potatoes were important to the war effort—*There's a war on!*

Beast was even worse the next morning. We stuck it out to the mid-morning break, then as a force-of-four, we told him that we'd complained to the Gaffer. Beast became angry. The four of us, as we had agreed before the break, clenched our fists and jutted our chins at him, and quit. Beast refused to drive us home, and told us to leave his property. We asked for pay earned. He refused to pay us for the two hours worked. Angry, penniless, and with no eggs to compensate, we made the five-mile trudge to Dunfermline. With no money, and no eggs to trade for bus fare from Dunfermline, we walked the remaining seven miles to Lochgelly. Our total transit from Beast's farm to home was more than five hours, including stops at private homes to beg water. Most unhappy, the Tattie Gaffer assigned us to closer and more tolerant farmers for the rest of the season. We never got paid for our two hours work, unless you count the half-dozen eggs we had purloined on our first day. We alerted our friends to Beast, but it's likely that other kids went to his distant farm. Much was allowed because, *There's a war on!*

I loved potatoes, everyway that my mum cooked them; thick cut sticks, deep-fried as chips, battered slices fried in pork lard as fritters; greased and roasted chunks in the oven while something else was cooking; boiled chunks served mashed with butter and salt; mashed chunks as a thickener in soups; chunks with rutabaga and carrots in a tasty soup—usually the vegetable chunks were our meal while Dad got the meat. In his physically demanding job of hewing coal, he got most of our family wartime meat and cheese rations. He needed protein, but did not get any extra rations.

The most wonderful potatoes I've ever eaten, absolutely, were cooked by myself, or by my friends, using a coal-fueled *fire-can*. Kids in my youth made fire-cans, and cooked potatoes in them. A dangerous method that we did well away from home—which was part of the fun. I made my fire-cans from an empty can, selected from a convenient rubbish bin, ideally about three inches in diameter and five inches tall. To admit air to enhance combustion, with a big nail and a rock, I punched holes in the bottom and halfway up the sides. Near the rim, I punched two holes to mount a bailing wire looped handle. With coal as a fuel, the can is a furnace. Whirled in a vertical loop at high speed, it becomes a blast furnace. A fire-can is good for only a few uses; the furious furnace effect destroys the can.

For those new to the art of fire-can cooking, newspaper and twigs are used to start a fire in the can, adding sticks as necessary. When the wood is ablaze, pieces of coal are added, and the can is whirled in a vertical loop. Then, more coal is followed by more can whirling till the furnace is smoke-free and the can, glowing red, is half-full of fiercely bright embers. That's when it's time to stuff a tattie (best snitched from a nearby field), ideally a skin-on Golden Wonder, about two inches across by three inches long, into the can. With a tattie securely in place, the fire-can is whirled to maintain a furnace-like temperature for maybe ten minutes—at least till the fire has charred the lower half of the tattie. Then, with a pair of sharp sticks, and risking blistered fingers, the potato is inverted, and the fire-can is whirled to cook the other half. With practice, a fire-can master can arrange to get one half of his *charrie-tattie* al dente, the other half pleasantly fluffy. They are wonderful hot, even without butter and salt; but do try the real treat—the black crust. With just the loose and flaky char rubbed off, a charrie-tattie crust is more than a tenth of an inch thick, with crunchy charcoal on the outside, and chewy chocolate brown on the inside—a gourmet treat! It also provides a fair dose of charcoal, considered by herbalists to be a beneficial toxin removal supplement for the body.

Grown-ups too, sometimes make *charrie-tatties* in the glowing embers of the open coal fires in their living rooms, perhaps to enjoy childhood taste-treats while forsaking the exciting dangers, imagine me: a braw wee Scotsman:

> In my ain cellar, wear'n a black velvet jaikit, and a kilt in the Robertson (Reid) hunting-tartan. Stood wi' ma back tae a toastin coal fire, I hautch ma kilt up . . ."Aye, it's a richt guid fire." A charring tattie is puffin a wee bit o' steam, and in ma left hand is a no well kent single malt Scotch, a three fingers splash—nae wat'r. My claymore hand is aye ready tae get the bottle fur a wee drap mair, while the tattie does its ain thing ben the guid fire. Doon ma stockin' leg, ma sgian dubh (stocking dagger) is ready tae cut the

charrie-tattie apart, but no yet, another wee drap or twa.

Reid (Red) is one of several septs of Clan Robertson of Struan, more properly called "Clan Dónnachaidh" (Don ah cah dee) children of Duncan I (1034–1040), King of Scots, a tragic character in Shakespeare's *Macbeth*). Another Duncan was a staunch supporter of King Robert the Bruce. In 1314, Duncan, led the Clan at the Battle of Bannockburn to victory over our great enemy, the *Sassenachs* (Saxons, now English). The Robertsons of Struan are the oldest documented clan in Scottish history, being the sole remaining branch of the Celtic Royal House of Atholl, which occupied the throne of Scotland during the 11th and 12th centuries, who in turn, were from a line of the kings of Dalriada in the 6th through the 8th centuries. Conan, the second son of Henry, the 3rd Earl of Atholl, inherited extensive lands. Other septs are: Collier, Duncan, MacConachie, MacIver, Roberts, and others. This little touch of heritage might explain some of my feelings about having to move from Scotland to England.

"Sassenachs! Go Live Among Them?"

I was seventeen in October 1947, when Dad decided to move our family from Lochgelly, in Fife (the peninsula with a Scotty dog profile on a map of east-central Scotland), to the Manchester area, in Lancashire, the economic center of Northwest England, and an epicenter of the Industrial Revolution that raged, like a virulent contagion, throughout the 1800's and early 1900's.

When Dad announced we were moving to the land of Sassenachs (Saxons), our traditional enemy, verse one of a popular pub song, *Bruce's March to Bannockburn* (Robert Burns), came to mind:

> Scots wha hae wi' Wallace bled
> *Scots wha' Bruce has often led,*
> *Welcome tae yer gory bed*
> *Or to victorie!*

The pastoral Kingdom of Fife was known in Pictish times as: *A right fair land and defendable peninsula,* and later, in 1050, was the capital from which the Celtic king, Malcolm III, ruled Scotland from the Royal Borough of Dunfermline—where his queen, Margaret, became a saint. The heart of King Robert the Bruce is buried in Dunfermline Abbey, along with other royalty and elite, and a small remnant of William Wallace, who was drawn-and-quartered by the Sassenachs. Andrew Carnegie, an American robber baron, and later, a generous philanthropist, was born in a weavers cottage in Dunfermline. In his youth, Carnegie was often hounded out of the magnificent Pittencrief estate (The Glen). He eventually purchased The Glen, and gave it, as Pittencrieff Park, to the people of Dunfermline. Seven miles by bus from Lochgelly, Dunfermline, its Glen, and its swimming baths, was one of my favorite haunts. Most of our relatives lived in or near Lochgelly, so did our many friends. Why did we move away from Fife?

In the summer of 1947, if there was a summer that year—nature skips Scotland now and then, my father forecast a decline of coal mining jobs in Fife. The Parliament in London was favoring the industrial areas of England with massive reconstruction funding for areas devastated by wartime air raids. Dad knew the coal fields in Lancashire wanted experienced miners. So, he got a job at a coal mine in Lancashire, living temporarily in a miner's hostel in Walkden in the heart of the mining region some 12 miles or so north of Manchester.

After some months, Dad came home to Lochgelly on a Friday night. He had a steady job, and was granted a mine-owned house to rent—a near miracle only two years after the war because housing was still in short supply. There had been no housing construction during those war years, and many homes were destroyed by German air raids. Dad told us the back of the house we were to live in faced the river Irwell, in the cotton-spinning and weaving town of Pendleton. He arranged for a friend who owned a coal delivery lorry (truck) to move us to Pendleton. Then he told us he would meet us at the Pendleton house in four weeks, and went back to Walkden the following afternoon.

The rest of the arrangements were Mum's responsibility. No small task, our move would be over more than 300 road miles from Lochgelly. I was seventeen and resourceful. My sister Jessie, fifteen, was a willing helper, but my brother Harry, just turned four, was a bit of a burden. We were to leave our *Happyland* tenement row house with a view of the Jenny Gray coal mine, and its busy and noisy chuff-chuff shunting locomotive, and move to a Pendleton house with a river view. It sounded wonderful, and as a keen angler, I was excited. But I was disappointed, too, at having to leave Moira, a 17-year old lass I had been courting for several months, and had been granted weekend living privileges at her mum's home. She lived in Blairgowrie, Perthshire, a 100-mile round trip bicycle ride. I had a last visit with Moira informing her, and her mother, that our budding affair was at an end. A mature young woman with a career in mind, Moira understood, because her dad, and her brother, like my dad, had found it necessary to work in England. They did construction work, but Moira's mum refused to move to Birmingham in England, choosing to live in their lovely home in Blairgowrie.

Dad warned us that we would have difficulty understanding the Lancashire folk. Odd, in that we laughed at, but understood the Scots talk and accents of Edinburgh, Glasgow and Perthshire, just as Moira and her family teased me with my *Fifer* talk. More a village than a town, Lochgelly was a backwater. The only foreign speaking people I had heard were during WWII. Free Polish soldiers, always chatty with our young women, would only say to us school kids, "*Nasdrovia*"; a greeting, or a killer scrabble word that meant, "Buzz off!" Perched on the highest land in Fife, Lochgelly had great views of Edinburgh across the Firth of Forth. Commando units from several nations trained on the steeper, firth side, of Lochgelly, on the Laird's country estate. The military sometimes barred us from going to the Loch, our favorite fishing and play area, which was also the Laird's property. We rarely saw any commandos. The few we did were not allowed to talk with us. It was "Hush-Hush," in WWII.

I remember having met only one English person before, and she had an incomprehensible cockney accent. Marjory appeared in my school class one day in early 1940. An evacuee from Blitz-ravaged London, she was blond and attractive, but naive about rural living and our way of talking. We kids called her "Margarine"— not for her hair color—margarine was the closest our accent matched how she pronounced her name— "Marjaree." She eventually stopped spelling out her name to us. By not bothering to learn her dialect, she had no choice but to learn ours.

Accent comprehension can be strange. We Fifers had no trouble understanding the talk in Hollywood movies, including the Movie-tone news clips, and comedy shorts such as the weekly showings of Shirley Temple, Our Gang (The Little Rascals), Abbot and Costello. Heck, we Scots even understood the weird lingo of Laurel and Hardy, and, of course, the accent-free body language of Charlie Chaplin, and Buster Keaton that lightened our sometimes weary lives.

Moving from Lochgelly meant breaking my contract as an indentured apprentice mechanic at the Nellie colliery and it could have been a legal issue. Fortunately (some investors would say unfortunately), in early 1947, all coal mines were nationalized, to be part of the National Coal Board (NCB), a government managed agency. The NCB enabled a transfer-continuation for

me to another coal mine within its national purview—
if an apprentice mechanic job was available. I quit the
Nellie coal mine with a week spare to help Mum pack.
Then, as often happens on moves, a two-week delay at
the Pendleton house made me a non-earner at a crit-
ical time when paychecks barely lasted a week. So I
got hired on as a day laborer to pick potatoes for two
weeks. Picking potatoes for six days a week earned me
almost four times as much as had my apprentice me-
chanic rate.

My feeling of loss at distancing relatives, friends,
and parting with Moira, was partly offset by the thrill
of moving to a strange land, strange as in unknown. I
had never been more than 60 miles from home. The
first time was during WWII, when my father's brother,
Jock, twice took me camping with his two sons to Bir-
nam Woods (think Macbeth), in Perthshire.

When the coal lorry that Dad had arranged for our
flit (move), came to our house in the afternoon before
the Saturday move day, we were packed, and the house
was scrubbed clean. I don't remember their names. I'll
call the driver Mac, and his helper, Don. The Coalman,
Mac, was freshly shaven, but looked like he had a blue-
black beard under his skin. He was a quiet man, about
the same height and build as my father. Dad had an
ideal miner's body; five-feet seven-inches tall, broad-
shouldered for his height, wiry looking, never an extra
globule of fat, rock hard muscles, steely-sinews, tortoise-
shell calluses, and tattooed from the waist up with the
dark-blue dashes and squiggles common to coal min-
ers. Miners rarely notice small cuts while working, or

if they notice, they just give the cut a quick rub to seal it with fresh coal dust. Freshly cut coal, fossil organics from the carboniferous age, is sterile. Healed cuts look like blue tattoos. The helper, Don, did not have a miner's build, but was tall and lanky. He had what was called a "lazy eye" and when he looked at you, it was a second or two before his left eye caught up with his good eye. Regardless, he was a carefree young man.

Mac and Don surveyed our belongings to decide how best to load the furniture. Our Happyland home had only two rooms, plus a small kitchen and an indoor toilet (no bath or shower), and was amply furnished with three double beds, a bulky easy chair (Dad's), a rocker (Mum's), a sideboard, a dining table with four chairs, a dresser, a tall wardrobe, rugs, and boxes of bits and pieces. Not much, but they were all of Mum's treasures. While the grownups sipped tea, discussed loading strategy, and a time of departure, I got the job of sweeping and cleaning the lorry. It was caked in coal-dust, and Mum was not going to put her precious things inside anything in such a filthy condition.

The eight-ton flatbed lorry with removable side railings used for our flit, necessitated a careful loading strategy before being draped with a tarpaulin for weather protection. Scottish weather, never predictable, is good for complexions, but deadly for lovingly polished wooden furniture. Mac and Don loaded most of the furniture that evening, leaving space on top for the two mattresses we were to use for our last night in Lochgelly. Then they arranged the tarp to make the lorry van-like, with the rear-flap open to load the mattresses, and as a balcony for Jessie and me to enjoy the journey.

It was still dark the next morning when Mac and Don loaded the mattresses, settled me in Dad's easy chair, and Jessie in Mum's rocker, our cruise accommodations, to look back at where we had been. Comfortably seated, Mum gave us cheese sandwiches and bottled tap water for the journey: then we heard the plan. To prevent unnecessary stops, Mac would park at public toilets, WC's (water closets), and whether we felt an urge, or not, we had to try. Mac, Don and I, would use the gentlemen's toilet—all three for the same penny in the slot. Mum, Harry and Jessie would do the penny routine in the ladies' toilet. Mum would be in the cab, with Harry perched on the seat, between her legs, occasionally spelled by Don; he liked kids. Mac, the only driver, was a smoker, and it was his lorry. Dad smoked. Mum never did. (Harry was the only one of their kids to smoke.)

Our journey was mostly experienced on poor grade roads. Like housing, roadway construction came to a halt during WWII. Roads in 1947 were mostly "B" rated or lower, quality "A" roadways were mostly still in the planning stages. On the early part of our journey, we headed west, just south of the Forth River, paralleling what was once the Roman Antonine Wall (143AD), that stretched from the Firth of Forth to the Firth of Clyde, the narrowest neck of land in Britain, The Antonine Wall proved ineffective at containing the barbarous Picts and was abandoned. A few hours later, near Carlisle (once one of five Roman Capital City's in Britain) we crossed the border into England—Sassenach territory. Near Carlisle, we passed a road-sign for the ruins of Hadrian's Wall (120AD). We had learned in school that the heavily fortified and garrisoned wall did keep the otherwise unconquerable Picts and Caledones at bay.

We enjoyed the sights of rich farmland and passing through quaint hamlets and villages. But not the congested towns and roadways crammed with noisy lorries that outnumbered cars, as we moved away from Scotland. By the late afternoon, we had sampled sunny, cloudy, and rainy weather, and had tasted Scottish mist, which we knew well. North English mist was much the same, as we neared Manchester, the mist tasted yucky—like pot-burned pea soup. It would get worse—confirming the reputation the industrial region of Lancashire had for being congested and cursed with a dismal climate.

Dad had told me that the Industrial Revolution, of which Manchester was a major hub, had long drawn the interest of many who had profited by ill-gotten gains from the Raj in India, the trading of opium to the Orient, and the transport of slaves to the United States. Such riches, invested in areas like Manchester, were blaringly trumpeted, as, "The Advancement of Civilization" "Prosperity Through Employment."

Many miles from Manchester, we entered a busy, buzzing, beehive world that was humming with the nectarous attractions of: coal mining; cotton spinning and weaving; machinery manufacturing, and the brewing of beer.

I soon found the investors were enlarging their fortunes from businesses spewing pollution and toxic waste, and requiring workers to toil long hours in dangerous working conditions. The abundance of beer breweries seemed necessary for the workers, as a throat rinse and palliative, especially for coal miners and cotton mill workers, laboring, nine-hour days, six-day weeks in contaminated atmospheres. Even those not employed, and workers after their labors, were affected by the polluted air and congested living conditions. I was not a beer drinker—my father drank my share. I managed with Vimto, a non-carbonated blackcurrant beverage.

Our arrival into the Greater Manchester area was a gloomy entry into a dank, industrial world—a soul-sinking experience. The most congested and noisy traffic we had ever experienced bumped ponderously around ugly, brick monoliths, with huge mine-buildings, massive cotton mills, windowless factories, and sudsy beer breweries. All had towering smokestacks, like a forest of prehistoric conifers sprouted from Carboniferous era seeds lurking in coal stored in their boiler bunkers, now grown 100 feet and more, aspiring odious mushroom canopies of sickly-brown, greenish-yellow, musty-gray misery. Adding to that were endless blocks of mill-owned and mine-owned, soot-stained brick row housing. Twenty or more homes in each tenement building, where every home had two or more coal-burning fireplaces. Graveyard-like rows of fancy clay chimneypots, poking above tenement roofs, were weeping ghastly greenish-yellow coal smoke. Leaden with sulfur and soot, seeping, lazily, down to ground level, the fumes were the reason, I thought, for the faint yellow tint in the stagnant air. Yet, more, as common as cockroaches, huffing coal-fired locomotives, puffing sulfurous geysers, were rumbling across rusted iron-bridges spanning over, and under us, bone-rattling cobblestone streets made talking impossible.

I was depressed, worried, scared! However, there were survivors. Pallid, ashen-like, expressionless faces, mostly men, wearing either brown or gray, flat, brimless caps, were sullenly gazing out of double rows of long grimy windows in the slab-like sides of large, cherry-red, double-deck buses—or were they ambulances? There were so many of them. At least the red double-deckers and gilded pub signs added color: not much else did. I saw streets with little old women, wearing crocheted shawls and long heavy skirts, in drab colors that were either a droll fashion mockery of the environment or camouflage. I noted them as gossiping neighbors of tenements that fronted onto many streets, their front doors separated from the cobblestone streets by only a four-feet wide flagstone sidewalk. The stoop, and sometimes the sidewalk in front of each door, was startlingly white from a practice I would come to know as *donkey-stoning*. Proud, or defiant, some housewives scrubbed the stone stoop and the concrete sidewalk with donkey-stone scouring blocks (available from rag and bone collectors). Some scrubbed daily, cosseting a hygienic extension of their home out into their circumscribed world, a chaotic world that poisoned even brick, stone and concrete. There was chaos in even thoroughfare and street arrangements, where grid plans were known only in other parts of the world. Our driver did not have a good map for the wilderness in which we were rambling, since Mac's originals were confiscated as a spy-thwarting measure in WWII, and he had yet to buy new ones. Signposts on major roadways had been replaced, but not yet the inner-city signs.

When off of the marked roads, Mac stopped often to get directions. The natives spoke a broad and oddly accented dialect, curiously complicated by their inability to sound "h's." I heard, "Turn right at the 'ospital, and 'ave a nice 'oliday." Mac patiently dealt with communication issues—dialect, accent, and slang—often discussed amid a quickly gathered, arm-waving crowd. It seemed that even the Sassenachs enjoy a Scots accent. The directions sometimes helped for a mile or less. Many street names changed in a fickle manner to something else, then back again, and the street nameplates played peek-a-boo with pub signs and mossy growth. The most effective directions involved pubs, because there was one on most every corner. Mac and Don learned to navigate, marine style, with waypoints provided by locals. "Ahead to the Giddy Sailor, starboard at the Golden Lion, ahead to the Brown Cow, port at the Chaucer's Arms, then ask anyone at the Skinny Maiden." Eventually, in the purple-tinted half-dark of twilight, we got precise directions to 60 Langley Road from a little old shawl-clad woman helping a limping dog across the street that even routed us to the correct side of the street for parking. As she advised Mac and Don, I saw the dog scamper away.

She was spot-on. We stopped in front of number 60 on a wide and busy street. It was a lovely house, a large two story semidetached (duplex), with sandstone windowsills, corbels, and door pillars, and a fancy wrought iron gate opening into a front garden of well-kept shrubs. I was tight behind Mac as he rang the doorbell, a ding-dong-ding chime. Pleased by the novelty, Mac tried a simple tune. A frowning old man wearing a shiny silk jacket opened the door, and I had a feeling he was not our butler. Dialect problems again were soon resolved with, slow and precise, proper English—gentry talk, from the peeved old man. He explained that we were on the wrong street, as his house was on Langworthy Road, while we sought Langley Road. More snooty-faced than earlier, the old man, aware of Langley Road as if he collected the rents there, gave Mac precise instructions, and added, "The pit houses," in what may have been his snootiest tone, "are just past the graveyard."

Without any other detours, Mac got us onto Langley Road, and quietly passed by the cemetery and its crematorium, then passed an acre or more of berry patch whose bramble stems, thicker than fat thumbs, were armed with life-threatening thorns. A narrow cinder-paved pathway separated the brambles from the pit-owned row houses. Mac stopped in front of the first building, a two-story 12-house tenement, one of four aligned on one side of Langley Road. Number 60 did not have a front gate, but did have a sliver of a front garden, enough for a single row of hardy marigolds. A definite downer, after thinking we had a stately semidetached with a gated front garden. The other side of the street was a block-long, noisy, toothpaste-tube manufacturing factory. It had many presses, each emitting one earth-trembling thump per toothpaste tube— awful for us as they operated 24 hours a day, but it was good for Jessie as she soon found a job there.

I knocked on the peeling paint. Dad opened the door, and as a tornado-driven straw might pierce a tree trunk, I lanced past him, knowing his eyes would be searching for Jessie and Harry, now that I was considered a man. This house was better, and larger, with four rooms instead of two. Downstairs was a kitchen, and two rooms, each with a coal-burning fireplace, with two bedrooms upstairs. Good, I thought, very good, but . . . ah . . . the toilet? I found it in the backyard, behind a red, wood-plank door—a phone booth sized shed—but with a proper flush toilet. What? Outside? Seven steps—rain or shine, maybe twelve when icy? No heater! Hmm—frostbite on tender skin might be a problem, but I soon got over that concern when I explored our long backyard. It had a sturdy gate, and a roomy shed that only used one end for coal storage. Wonderful! Most of this shed will be for my bicycle and my workshop.

Our only toilet being outside was a downer, but I decided our new home was, overall, a definite plus. It was too dark to see the river Irwell, and I had to help unload the lorry. Dad's easy chair and Mum's rocker were first to be taken off, then the dining set. Dad had got food in, and Mum was soon cooking bangers (pork sausages) with mashed potatoes and tinned (canned) peas. That first meal in our new home tasted wonderful, and gave us energy for the work still to be done. Unloaded and assembled, the beds were made ready with sheets, blankets, and quilts. Everyone was ready for sleep, but not until the lorry was emptied, and everything set in the house, some randomly. Then, I had my first night's sleep in Sassenach territory, temporarily sharing a bed with Jessie. In bed, I thought, tomorrow morning—the river—something old-snoot-face on Langworthy Road doesn't have.

From the upstairs back bedroom window, in the gray of morning light, I saw wisps of mist rising from the Irwell, and saw that we were on a plateau, about forty feet higher than the river. The river looked wide. I knew from a library book that the Irwell fed into the 36 miles of the Manchester Ship Canal, an engineering triumph that made the inland cities of Manchester and Salford ports for large freighters that plied the world via Irish Sea access. I dressed quickly and dashed down to the near bank. Heartbreak. Damn! The Irwell was grossly polluted! With raw sewage, industrial effluents, and coal dust as fine as facial makeup. The water was opaque black, with creamy foam where roiled by occasional turbulence, much like a freshly poured pint of Guinness stout. But it was a toxic brew, and Guinness has a tolerable smell.

Although difficult to believe, the following June I watched, amazed, a Rowing Regatta on the sudsy Irwell. An annual rivalry that involved the two Manchester Universities: each fielding Eights with Coxswain: Twos: and Single Sculls. Starting at Salford College, well downstream from our home, the crews rowed upstream on a placid but turbid course. Passing our home, and the rear of Salford Cemetery, to a finish at the Agecroft Road Bridge, near the ever-scented Cuzzons soap and perfume works. The popular footpath on the Langley Road side of the Irwell was lined with spectators. The other side, downwind of the prevailing breeze, had no footpath, just dozens of soccer, rugby and cricket fields. Perhaps because both universities had famous medical schools, I never saw the traditional ritual of dumping the Eights-coxswain in the river. The rowers natty white outfits may have been disposable, perhaps also their craft and oars.

I later learned that new sewage plants and effluent controls, delayed by WWII, were again under construction. After a few years, the river became sewage and effluent free. It lost its creamy cap, but it remained black for some years after the mines closed in the 1980's. (In July 2005, I walked the Irwell footpath, still a lover's lane, but now graced by the clear water of the Irwell, where anglers again catch fish.)

After our first breakfast in Langley Road, Mum found a problem—her galvanized iron pail for cleaning floors and suchlike, was missing. All shops were closed on Sundays in 1947. So my mum managed with a large enameled-steel *po* (Fife), a *goesunder* (Lancashire), *a chamber pot* to the prim old geezer on Langworthy road. Dad sketched directions for a shortcut to an ironmonger (hardware shop), where I was to go on Monday to buy a six-gallon pail. Early Monday morning, I set off along the remnants of an old road, crossed two soot-blackened, iron bridges spanning over a railway and a sorry looking, algae-blanketed canal. Then I hurried across an active refuse dump, and hustled up a hilly street to the village of Ir'lam o'the Height's (high above the Irwell).

Soon after 9:00 a.m., I was asking a gray-eyed, ruddy-jowled, red-veined nose, old Lancastrian for a pail. Was his blank stare a message? Is he deaf? Slower, I asked again, and received the same response, except he shifted his weight to the other foot. I asked, in my best Lochgelly *pan-loafie* (formal) tongue, then watched his brows narrow as he shook his head, slow enough to not risk injury or disturb the few wisps of white hair on his balding pate. He spread an arm expansively. That, I understood, so I browsed the randomly scattered goods in his store—without success. I answered his expectant look by saying, "Pail," spelling "P-A-I-L," and hand-gestured what I thought suggested a pail, and noted his sloth-like shrug and vacant gaze. With nary a word, he turned on his steel-shod, wooden-soled, clog-clad feet, and carefully plopped to the back of the shop and on into his humble home. The plop step, I learned when I wore clogs for almost a year, was devised to lessen the clatter made by clogs worn by many workers in Lancashire.

Ruddy Jowls returned with a short, stout, and comely old woman, dressed, of course, in standard Lancashire dress and camouflage colors, and even indoors she was wrapped in a beige crochet shawl. I returned her sweet smile, spelled, "P-A-I-L," in pan-loafie while repeating my hands-as-pail pantomime. Her blue eyes flashed and then sparkled as she turned to Ruddy Jowls. I didn't understand her gentle words. His explosion of what might have been words also energized him.

With arms swinging, Jowls clattered his clogs to a closet, and with dry hinges whining, opened its double doors—treasure shone bright—two, new, gleaming, galvanized iron pails. I grabbed the larger one. Ruddy Jowls, in his, "another-satisfied-customer" voice, in what I would later learn was Ir'lam o'the Height's dialect, narrowed and slowed for my foreign ears, said, *"Eee lad, tha wont's a blody booket."* I sensed booket, might be bucket. When he repeated his utterance, I translated it, "Young man, you want a bloody bucket." Simple: after I surmised bucket, and realized that *blody* meant bloody—a gentle swear word throughout the British Isles.

Perhaps because of Bannockburn, Ruddy Jowls charged more than I expected for the pail, or he added a translation fee, or an extra for a primer in *o'the Height's* dialect. Always pleased to see me on later visits to his shop, he called me *Schochy.* I thought of him as *Yokel.* I only went to him for convenience; elsewhere cost less—thrifty Scots mind such matters. It has forever bothered me that Yokel didn't understand plain-as-print, Fife pan-loafie.

My Lancashire wife, Tessa, enjoys telling people about my accent issues, especially my pail episode. And of her experience in Fife, learning from my aunt the proper use of pan-loafie: a Fife metaphor: "As formal as pan loaves," which is bread baked in a closed pan so that it has a perfect brick-like shape and all surfaces have a uniformly thin crust. Bread preferred by those of genteel mien or social standing—like the silk-jacketed geezer—but not Yokel.

In the afternoon of the pail affair, I went with Dad by bus to the NCB head offices in Walkden. There I presented my Indenture and asked to resume my apprenticeship. Regardless of my colliery experience, the NCB enrolled me in a two-week mining orientation course, compulsory for all hires and all job classes. In my case, with almost four years of coal mine experience—an obvious waste of money—a common fault with the government run NCB. I knew more than the course leader, and on the first morning, he made me his assistant. Pan-loafie was working for most of the attendees. Word of my knowledge got back to those that mattered. Right from the orientation course, I was hired as an apprentice mechanic at the Wheatsheaf Colliery, in Pendlebury, a town next to Ir'lam o'the Height's. Getting to the Wheatsheaf was a thirty-five-minute walk, or an easy bicycle ride—except for Icky Brew, a steep road made slippery with copious pigeon droppings (icky) splattered on coarse cobblestones.

When I resumed my apprenticeship at the Wheatsheaf Colliery in Pendlebury in 1947, it would be three years before I learned that Tessa Gallagher lived in Pendlebury, and that she worked as a bookkeeper at Cuzzons, the soap and perfume works near Langley Road. And interestingly, my Scots accent issues at the Wheatsheaf, and my interest in bicycling, were factors, in 1950, that influenced Tessa Gallagher, a Sassenach, to ask her brother-in-law to suggest that I be her blind date for the November 13 annual Policemen's Ball, a date we still celebrate.

Tessa and I married in March 1952, and emigrated from England in 1956 with our three-year old son, Grahame. Wearing his kilt, sporran and tweed jacket, Grahame, on the Cunard Franconia, and for three days in New York, was the darling of many, often lifted and hugged by many an Irish policeman. We settled in Monrovia, California. On Pearl Harbor Day, December 7, 1957, we proudly welcomed an American into our family, our daughter, Helen.

Back in England, the killer fogs and unhealthy air improved when Greater Manchester converted to smokeless-fuel, coke—coal baked at a high temperature to extract valuable chemicals. Many years later, on our trips from California to visit relatives in Britain, strikingly, everywhere, but particularly in the Greater Manchester area, the blackened sandstone of churches and other magnificent architectural buildings had gradually healed back to natural creams, grays, tans, pinks and pale-reds. Convenient truths are that controlling pollution encourages nature to heal. And that Sassenachs are worth getting to know.

With over fifty-seven years of marriage to Tessa, Burns's pan-loafie, from *O My Luve's Like a Red, Red Rose,* speaks for me:

> As fair art thou, my bonie lass
> So deep in luve am I,
> And I will luve thee still, my dear
> Till a' the seas gang dry.

Joanne Simpson

Reading Joanne's memoirs, one thinks of the great tragic women of literature: Anna Karenina, Emma Bovary, Tess of the d'Urbervilles. Of course, one of the joys of the senior citizens' writing workshops is learning of the triumphs and tragedies of the participants' lives. Joanne's stories need only more texture and depth to make them into memorable literature—but that's the case with every life story: the framework, the raw material is there, to be developed.

One distinction we make is that between "chronicle" and "history." A chronicle is a record, a history is a story. Anyone can write a chronicle, and I think that anyone can write a history, given the will to do so and rich feedback from readers.

—W.R.W.

Bubbles of Remembrance

As bubbles blown into the air
Float and shimmer with rainbow colors,
Then, abruptly, burst into nothingness;
So do memories spark into my mind,
Colorfully linger as a picture show,
Then, suddenly, vanish from consciousness.

It Was the 60's!

Nineteen sixty-six in the San Francisco-Oakland area was the *back to nature* era of hippies, peace signs, flowers-in-the-hair, Tree People; make-your-own-bread/jellies/pies/beads/clothes; *free love,* topless bars, Go-Go dancers; *End-the-War* liberals vs. the John Birch Society ultra conservatives in our Walnut Creek neighborhood.

I had quit teaching my high school job. With a young daughter, directing plays, coaching speech tournaments, teaching English to freshmen, sophomores, and seniors, I was just gone too much, and, when home, I was correcting papers and making lesson plans. Something felt wrong, like my child was being cheated. Though she had a wonderful baby sitter, none of us were ever home! We had moved from Southern California to further Bob's career, but he often had late meetings with a long commute everyday. Though the money was helpful, I felt that I could be a full-time homemaker and mom, thus saving the need for a baby sitter, a housekeeper, and a gardener. And, I could substitute teach a couple of days a week. (The pay was $17.00 a day!)

Bad move!

One evening, as I was baking bread, I answered the phone.

"Is this Bob's wife?" a woman's voice asked.

"Yes, who is this?" I answered.

"Well, it doesn't matter, but I wanted you to know that I'm upset that Bob is dancing with someone else.

He usually dances with me! I thought you should know (sobbing a bit)—in case you're divorcing soon!" Click!

What was going on? I was usually asleep when he'd have late meetings, but had I been asleep to the kind of *meetings* he'd been having? Was I so trusting and naïve that I hadn't even noticed that he'd strayed, or was it all some cruel joke? He hadn't taken me out dancing in ten years. He hated to dance! He'd always complain that we were spending too much money, so we rarely went out to dinner, unless it was with a client and wife.

It was very late when he got home, so he was surprised to see that I was awake.

I asked, "How was the meeting? Where was it? Who all was there?"

He was evasive, saying, "Oh, you don't know them. It was at an office in San Francisco. It didn't go too well, so I'm extremely tired!"

Obviously, he didn't know the gal had called. I was livid! I related the message to him—word-for-word.

Bob was hardly ever at a loss for words, but that night, he was. I could almost see his mind searching for something to say. His face and neck got red. He tried to speak, gave it up, and, grabbing his coat, just walked out! The front door slammed, and I heard the car starting up. He was gone.

Most of this time remains a blur. I was stunned.

Trying to make sense of the whole mess, we met with our minister, but not much help there, since he only instilled a lot of guilt in both of us.

"Where is your husband staying? Aren't you worried?"

"No, I don't really know or care."

"Bob, don't you miss your home and daughter?"

Silence.

Though Bob would not, I visited a recommended psychotherapist. He gave no clue of how to begin, or what to say. I sobbed. He said, "It's your hour." Without guidelines, I just cried the time through, and went home. Some help! I then saw a psychiatrist, a father of one of my former students. He asked questions, listened, and then said, "Well, I would say that you shouldn't have married each other in the first place!" Big help that was—my family had told me that! (Of course, because they'd been against it, we had stubbornly gone ahead and planned our own wedding!) Well, so much for expensive treatment *of the id by the odd!*

At least Bob and I were talking—sort of. He was terribly unhappy. Our sex life had never been *fireworks.* Since we'd both been *virgins,* I guess I had just chalked it up to that Peggy Lee song, *Is That All There Is?* and gone on with my life. I had not ever thought of straying, or if something was missing in marriage. Back in the 50's, one did not marry to be divorced!

In the meantime, I'd tried to get a full-time job again. Wrong timing! None of the school districts was hiring. I certainly couldn't keep the house on a sub's pay. Since Bob had always handled financial matters, I wasn't sure how bad things were. The only place that wanted to hire me was a Catholic high school in Vallejo. Someone needed me! However, the drive was across the county and over the bay bridge, and the pay was two-thirds less. No way could that cover house payments, let alone child care costs. I did office jobs—temporary Kelly Girls assignments in local businesses and stores. I continued to substitute as often as possible for four different districts. Once, I even subbed in Oakland's Youth Incarceration Center. I didn't know if my high school students were just runaways or murderers. I entered the classroom with the supplies (but no pens or pencils—nothing *sharp*), and the door was locked behind me! I don't even remember what I was supposed to teach, so I think I mainly just read to them. I'm sure it wasn't memorable to them, either. I never went back.

The Continuation School in Walnut Creek called to say they needed a long-term sub. This was the district's high school for those students who, for one reason or another, were failing regular school. In most cases, it was not due to stupidity, but family problems, drugs, and probation matters were the usual culprits for their schooling here. Joe, a wonderful principal, had known me from my previous job, so he sat me down and explained this job. The regular teacher was hospitalized, but was expected to return in about six weeks. Joe said, "I know you, Joanne, and I fear you are going to be taken in by these kids. I know you can teach, but I want to warn you not to believe them in most instances. They'll try to con you, so you can't be too soft with them. Many have drug problems, and some have records of theft. Some will break your heart with their stories." Well, since my heart was already broken, I could see no difficulty.

I taught only three classes, with five to fifteen students in the morning and seven in the afternoon. It was one of the few campuses in California to have a smoking section. Since I was smoking then, and most of my students were, too, we even had breaks together. Most of the curriculum was already set up so that I only arranged it to fit the kids' interest (or, lack of) in English and Social-Studies. By the end of the first week—we were reading and discussing the novel, *Airplane*—I had worked up a word puzzle and quiz, made them copies, and passed them out to the students on Friday. What a shock! They looked at me in amazement, started folding the papers, and proceeded to *fly* my *Airplane* dittos around the room. Even *Peaceful Paul*—so named because he was usually quiet, wore the hippy peace sign, and spouted Biblical messages of peace—turned his table on its side, and pretended to machine-gun down the paper airplanes!

Maureen, a particularly friendly student, saw my surprise and took me aside, saying, "We don't work on Fridays!"

"Oh," said astonished me. "What do you do?"

"We usually just talk, or draw."

"Thanks. So, is there anything wrong today, Maureen? You look like you've been crying."

She laughed, "Oh, no. It's just the marijuana. Didn't you know it makes your eyes red?" No. I hadn't known that . . . or, lots of other things that those kids taught me. One day, Tim came late to class. He had been absent for three days. I asked him if he was feeling all right, if he'd been sick. He steered me to one side of the room, confided that he'd been arrested, and wondered if I could speak on his behalf at his trial. I think I stammered out something about not being allowed to do that. I asked him what had happened. His story involved his *needing* drugs . . . receiving them, and not being able to pay . . . involved with a burglary . . . but, he "didn't know the guy had guns" . . . getting caught, he "didn't know about the drugs in the truck where they'd put the stolen goods!" Poor Tim. He never returned. How I wish I could have helped him—somehow—someway!

On campus we had a deputy sheriff assigned to the school who knew most of the students. Sometimes we'd chat at lunch or recess, and discuss various things. I was surprised to learn that he knew of my separation and possible divorce. I really had not told many people, including my own family! If my students saw me talking to the deputy, they'd just shake their heads, *no,* and turn away. I assumed they were afraid I'd tell him secrets about them.

I said to Maureen, "I would never divulge any information about any of you. Why did you shake your finger, *no,* when I was speaking to him today?"

She replied, "Do not ever trust that man! He does terrible things to kids. Don't ever tell him anything about yourself!" I thought she was just talking about students being arrested for their illegal acts.

But my job there was soon finished, because their regular teacher was returning.

One day on the way home, I stopped at the hardware store. As I was checking out, I saw that same deputy sheriff. We smiled, said "Hello," and I went to my old Rambler station wagon. He came after me, flashed his badge, and he said I was under arrest.

"What?—What are you talking about?" I asked, thinking it was a joke.

"I saw you take those two items after you checked out," he replied.

"Which items? I have my receipt," I answered, trying to figure out what he was saying. He grabbed my wrist, took my bag of items, and marched me back into the store to a side office. He called in the manager, showed him a pair of large white Bermuda shorts (clearly not my size 8), and a huge tee shirt, that were in my basket, and not paid for. The police were called. They drove me, shocked and sobbing to the police department. I couldn't believe what was happening. Had I totally flipped out? I couldn't remember where those things were in the store, let alone taking them! I felt like I was in a nightmare, as I was fingerprinted, photographed, then released to go home. I would be informed, they explained, when to appear in court!

Driven back to my car, I somehow was able to get my daughter from the sitter, and drive home. As I fixed her dinner, she knew something was wrong. We went to bed early. Numbly, crying, I tried to piece together what had happened. How had I done this? How would I ever be able to face neighbors, friends, family, again? When had I shoplifted? Why would I? The bottom of my stomach lurched. My teaching credentials! I would never be able to teach again. How could I make a living for my daughter and me? Would I be put in jail? What would happen to her? I couldn't think. I couldn't sleep. I couldn't breathe!

The next day, a Saturday, I drove my daughter to a friend's house for the day. Returning home alone, I didn't really know what I was going to do. The doorbell rang. Answering the door, I saw that Deputy Sheriff. He said he was so sorry about what had happened, and he said that he felt he could help me. I invited him in, asked if he'd like some coffee. As I headed to the kitchen, he followed, asking, "Do you have a tape recorder?"

"No. Do you need one? I can borrow a neighbor's," I replied.

"No, no. That's okay. Nice house. Anyone else home?"

"No. Not right now."

"Let's see the rest of your place. Nice bedroom," he said as he walked toward it. "How do these drapes close?"

Oh, no! The light dawned!

"They don't! You'd better leave—Now!" I sternly sputtered, finally realizing what was going on. Walking quickly to the front door, I stepped out and held it for his exit. My heart was racing. Was he going to pull a gun? What could I do now? Which neighbors were home? Who'd believe me?

He calmly sauntered out, saying, "You just made a big mistake!" Getting into his white official car, he drove off.

I stood there, shaking. Just then, Bob drove up. "Was that a county car that just left? Who was visiting?"

Tears welling up, my face must've been drained of color, as I told him what had been going on. He seemed to be confused, comforting, outraged, too. (Later on, I wondered, had Bob been in on it? Was it a set-up?)

The next week, we saw our lawyer, the one we'd hired origally for a divorce. Bob said that he wanted to come home, and try to work things out. We both asked the lawyer to check on that deputy to see what could be done about his actions. I wanted him to be arrested, and taken away from the high school. I finally realized what Maureen had been trying to tell me. What horrible things had he done to students, too scared to tell on him—and, who could they tell? Who would believe them?

My lawyer replied, "And, who will believe you? I'll check on him, but I want to warn you, you're just a substitute teacher! You were arrested! You're going through a divorce! This could turn out ugly, and you'll lose your credentials. Think of the publicity and your daughter."

What a shock! Upon investigation, the deputy was found to be an upstanding citizen with a wife and four children, residing in a nearby town. I was devastated to learn he was never questioned by the authorities.

My lawyer cleared matters with the court, so the shoplifting charges were dismissed. Upon the receipt of a questionnaire from the State of California Credentials Committee, he responded for me, and my record was cleared. Whew!

Bob came home, but things did not get better. I'd been taking birth control pills, which were new on the market. We didn't want any mistakes! The pills did not agree with me, and I often got crying jags. Bob thought I was just hysterical!

One late night, Bob called to say that he had just saved someone from jumping off the Bay Bridge, and was going to get a hotel room for them. I said to bring him home, that we could help him here, but he replied that *she* wouldn't want to do that. I could see the hand-writing on the wall that he was messing around again. I was livid when he got home the next day. I asked him what's going on, and he said he wanted to leave. I in-sisted that he explain that to our daughter, but I knew it was best that he just go!

I stopped the pills—no more crying! I really wasn't *nuts* after all!

Later that week, while waiting in the center lane at a stoplight, an old, dirty, *peace-scrawled* van zoomed to a stop next to me. Like huge, unkempt ants, kids swarmed out and ran over to my car. They were *My* kids—from the Continuation High School.

Smiling, they said, "Hi! We've missed you!"

"Is this your daughter?"

"She's so cute!"

"When can you come back?"

The people in the cars around us sat stunned with wide-eyed, shocked expressions, not knowing if a gang was attacking me. I put the car in park, got out, and hugged each one, saying, "We're on the way home. Want to come by?"

It was then that I received the most unusual compli-ment of my teaching career:

"Oh, no! We couldn't do that!"

"Why not?" I asked. "It's not far from here."

"Cause, you see, we really like you. And, we'd be casing your place, and we just wouldn't ever want to steal from you!" Jim explained. And, waving, they were gone; my sweet, *honest* kids!

No husband. No job. No home . . . I knew then that I had to call my mom and sis, and move my daughter and me back to Southern California to find a job. So, scraping myself together, and putting on my *smiley face*, I did just that!

Fred

I'd finally met HIM—The Man of My Dreams—Love of My Life—My Future. After two disastrous marriages, many dates, several affairs, he was *The One*. Of course, I was already 66 years old! Let me tell you how we met.

It isn't easy being single in a couple's world. Joining the Crystal Cathedral Singles Group, I had met many nice people, especially women with whom I could bond. This group was, and still is, so friendly, caring, and fun. We're a diverse bunch, most of us over fifty, female, and empty-nesters. I had noticed Fred, because he always seemed to be on the outskirts of any meeting, with his shirts kind of rumpled and younger than most of us. Polite, smiling, but not really joining in with the rest, unless called on. He'd been a member for several years, though absent a lot. Soon, we got to talking, and we realized that we both had the same, rather cynical, *Mad Magazine* type of humor.

Whenever someone asked, "Hi, Fred, how are you?"

He'd always answer, "Mean, rotten, nasty, and cruel."

Of course, he was just the opposite.

We enjoyed each other's company whenever we were both at meetings on Tuesday nights, or Sundays, after which we'd all go out to brunch. I kept looking for a gal for Fred. He was educated, fun, nice-looking, and very intelligent. He had so much knowledge about so many different things. He said he had a head full of trivia: nothing that was useful. Ask him about U.S. history, he could tell you the dates of battles, or who was President, when, and name the Vice-President, too. I thought he should go on *Jeopardy*. He would just laugh and say that as an auditor-accountant, he just naturally remembered numbers and facts.

I noticed that when a waiter would bring the bill, Fred had already figured it out—to the penny—adding a generous tip. Well, that impressed me, because I am definitely math dyslexic!

I knew that he had had a bad marriage, a bitter divorce, three children, and one step-daughter. His only son lived with him. So, he wasn't looking for a wife and family, just companionship. He was rather gun-shy about any commitments, and none of the ladies his age seemed to be his type.

One time we all went to eat at a *Benihana* restaurant, and Fred asked if he could buy me lunch. Realizing that he was just being polite and probably could not afford it, I declined. "But, I'd enjoy sitting with you," I added.

"What, are you crazy?" friend Bob remarked. "Here's a guy who says he'll buy!"

Fred just grinned, but I think he was relieved. I'd never gotten the hang of using chopsticks, so Fred was demonstrating picking up objects while we waited for the food. Using them, he pointed out the metal clamps used instead of buttons on the suit I was wearing. He asked, "How do these undo?"

I replied, "Well, you're so adept with the chopsticks, you might figure it out."

He actually blushed.

After a potluck dinner at Christmas, he helped me carry some things to my car. Our two old red cars were parked side by side. In unison, we said, "See, red's my favorite color!" I mentioned that he hadn't danced much, and there were a few young women he hadn't asked. He replied, "I like the one with the old, red car." I couldn't believe that he preferred this old lady.

We became good friends, and looked forward to seeing each other at get-togethers. His dry sense of humor, quick wit, true wisdom of subject matter (including the Bible), and funny redneck jokes livened any subject. He was showing up more often, and I was still searching for a date for him—though not as vigorously.

One evening, my friend had tickets to a ballet at the Performing Arts Center, and asked if I'd like to take her place, as she couldn't go. "Oh, yes!" I replied. Fred overheard, and asked if he could join me. I was amazed.

This man liked classical music and stage shows, too! Great! We met at a nearby restaurant first, ate, and leaving my car in the parking lot, we walked to the theatre. It was a stunning performance. He'd parked his car at the Center, so he drove me back to my car. I couldn't find my keys. Oh, no! Where were they? At the show? In the restaurant? It was closed! However, one of the waiters was just getting to his car. Fred flagged him down and the two of them yelled their way in. Fred zoomed out a side door, triumphantly waving my keys. I'd lost them on the floor under our table. What a relief! I was so embarrassed.

"My hero!" I exclaimed, kissing him on the cheek.

He hugged me and said, "I haven't been kissed in seven years."

I replied, "Seven years is too long!"

He smiled and quipped, "Silly me, I should've hidden the keys, and said you'd just have to come home with me, that we'd find them tomorrow."

By October, we were e-mailing jokes to each other, and we talked on the phone a few times a week. The Sunday before Columbus Day, Fred said he had Monday off, and wondered if I'd like to go for a ride. Of course I did. He drove us to Ports-O-Call, and we walked around, talking about our growing up here in Southern California (he was a true *prune-picker*—a native Californian). We shared our backgrounds, good times, and sad ones, too.

"How about some merlot?" Fred asked as he spied a restaurant.

"I've never tried it, but I'd like to," I replied, sitting opposite him at the table.

The waiter brought the wine in tall, thin-stemmed glasses. I was describing something, with my usual wild hand gestures, when I knocked over my glass of merlot—onto Fred's lap.

"Oh, no! I'm so sorry. Let me help you!" I yelled . . . inadvertently hitting my glass of ice water, right on top of his wine-soaked shirt and pants.

"Yikes!" was his surprised yelp, as he jumped up. "You could've just told me that you don't like merlot— or, is it me?"

I apologized profusely. He ordered more wine for me and suggested they bring it in a mug! I felt so badly; he was very gracious. We laughed, I offered to get his clothing dry-cleaned. He said, "No, but a kiss would be nice."

Of course, I complied. Thus ended, our first date. I then bought him a pair of stain-resistant, wrinkle-free pants and a shirt! We've had many more *Merlot Mondays*.

Actually, sixteen years difference in age is a lot! That he was the younger bothered me, but it didn't faze Fred. Since he had three older sisters, he couldn't see any problems and got agitated if I mentioned it. However, he did decide to grow a full beard (to look older, perhaps?). Our friends and families thought that we were close enough in thought, ideas, looks, attitudes, likes and dislikes, if not in years. After all, he was the one with the silver-threaded, dark brown hair. Mine was still gray free. I said we were the *Ashton Kutcher-*

Demi Moore of the geriatric group. (Fred didn't think that was funny.)

Standing five-feet, nine inches tall, with a slightly chubby build, my four-feet eleven inches fit just right under his arm. Glasses covered his soft green eyes, but his mischievous twinkle gleamed. Through four years, we lived and loved, and enjoyed each other so much. However, we really had only weekends together, mostly at my place. When Fridays came, he'd arrive after work. I'd hear a loud "MEOW" under the kitchen window and say, "Oh, oh, it's that old Tom Cat again. I wonder what he wants!" At the door, a bouquet of flowers would appear, and Fred would arrive with chocolate, or wine, or ice cream, and swoop me up in hugs and kisses. Oh, and he'd always remember to bring treats for my cat—who loved Fred, too! We'd have appetizers and wine, chatting while I'd fix dinner. We actually would eat in bed on lap trays, watching Jeopardy on TV, amazed and laughing at our intelligent (or not!) answers. Quite often, we never made it to Wheel of Fortune, because we were each other's dessert. Physically, our union grew in passion: anxiously exploring each other, my skin tingling at his touch. He would kiss my toes and other places! We would melt into heart-pounding, delicious sex.

Saturdays and Sundays became my never-before-experienced *honeymoons*. We'd take road trips, traverse museums, see movies, symphonies, or stage shows, dine out, then fall asleep wrapped together, his body always so warm and comforting.

During this time, Fred's son, Jon, who was used to sitting in the front seat with his dad, was delegated to the back of the car—not exactly to his liking. He had graduated from high school, but still hadn't passed his driver's test ("Why bother, when I don't have a car?" he would say.), hadn't enrolled in college, nor gotten a job. Though Fred was proud of his son, Jon became a source of worry and hurt to Fred. Jon knew how to *push his buttons.* Just to threaten that he would leave, as Fred's other children had, would wound Fred's heart. Having divorced a money-grabbing, non-working, conniving wife, and sometimes working three jobs, Fred had gone through major depression, losing his home, job, health, and future. (Of course, I only know his side, but I believe him.) His sisters came to his rescue. The family had never liked his wife, and all knew how hard Fred had tried to keep his family together. With help, Fred got healthier and landed a secure job. Then, he discovered that Jon's mom was making Jon, at age fifteen, live in the garage. When she kicked him out, Fred filed for and got full custody. Jon's mom remarried and moved away, so the girls all decided to move in with their Dad—bringing a young grandson and a dog, too. Squashed into a small apartment, Fred's paycheck just couldn't cover five dependents, and no one else would get a job, or do the housework, laundry, shop, cook, or even walk the dog! Soon, Fred said they'd have to find employment. The girls resisted; Fred insisted. So, his step-daughter called the police, yelling into the phone, "He's hurting us!" The police arrived. Fred was humiliated. What a mess! By the time all was straightened out, the girls found jobs (or boyfriends) and moved out. Regardless, Fred was to have no contact with them (though that was not a court order; they were all over twenty-one). Fred has missed his grandson . . . and the dog.

Of course, this was all so hurtful, and took a toll, physically and emotionally. When Jon couldn't get his way with Fred—wouldn't go to college, do housework, laundry, shopping, get a job, or go to counseling, all Jon had to do was hint about leaving, and Fred would fulfill Jon's wishes. Though he really couldn't afford to, he would buy Jon buying new video games, computer games, Direct TV, or new cards to play *Lord of the Rings* tournaments. Fred would drive Jon and friends to Las Vegas, San Diego, or other places to play these games—it was costly!

As a single mom, I had participated in what I call *The Single Parent-Child Game*, trying to do everything for my fatherless daughter. By the time Fred realized what the game was, too, with his own son, we had been seriously dating. Needless to say, Jon, didn't care much for me.

Fred's sisters and brothers-in-law, however, did. They knew how happy Fred and I were, how we helped each other with problems, how we enjoyed being together. They'd include me in all family celebrations, and we'd join them on vacations or get rooms with their timeshares. When one sister, Joan, and husband, Tom, moved to Seattle, Fred's other sister, Mabel, her husband, Louis, Fred and I, took a wonderful vacation trip to visit them. Since they, too, are intelligent, educated, loving people, we like many of the same things. Just last fall, taking my new red Honda Accord (which Fred had helped me pick out and get financing for), we toured the Redwoods, the Oregon coast, Washington, and Vancouver. Crossing the glass-bridge in Redding, visiting state capitols and monuments, hiking through the wondrous forests, admiring the waterfalls, rocks, flowers, seascapes, lighthouses, and farmland scenery, then, celebrating Tom's eightieth birthday with friends and relatives. We had a great time!

Until on our way home, we got into stop-and-go-traffic in Sonoma, California. Fred was driving, and we had come to a complete halt. I just happened to glance at the side view mirror, when I saw this truck, barreling down on us.

"Oh, no!" I yelled. "He's not going to"—CRASH!

The truck slammed into us. That truly shook us up! Cell phone calls resulted in the CHP, police, and an ambulance's arrival. No one was badly hurt, just my car, with a caved-in trunk. We were lucky. (Could that be because Louis is a minister? Or, because we had so much luggage in the trunk it cushioned the blow?) However, the trunk lid wouldn't close. Because it was a Saturday afternoon, 5:30, the Auto Club couldn't get us to an open repair shop. So, Fred tied it down, using his shoelaces. (Ingenious, huh?) Knowing it wouldn't hold for very long, we slowly drove into town. I spied a motorcycle shop that looked as if someone was still inside, and jumped out to check, while Fred parked the car.

I called out, and a loud, gruff voice answered, "We're closed!"

I went around to the back gate, and this huge, tattooed biker loomed in front of me.

"Wait. We need your help. Do you have a bungee cord we could buy to hold our damaged trunk?" I stammered.

Just then, Fred zoomed to my side, holding up a twenty-dollar bill. When Mr. Grouch realized we were in trouble, and came out to look. Since he'd locked up, he couldn't get back into the building. Just then, Big Baby Biker roared up on his Harley. He had a roll of duct tape. Well, that worked, and we drove off, taped together with that twenty dollar roll of silver duct tape. With a big silver X taped across the trunk's lid, attached to each side of the car, and to the bumper, it held the dangling license plate and kept the trunk lid from flying up.

There just aren't any vacant motel rooms during the summer on a Saturday night. We were way behind schedule, Fred was exhausted, and his sister was still recovering from a recent eye surgery. Since they would only hold the rooms at our next motel destination for two more hours, we had to keep driving, over the bridge through the San Francisco traffic, stopping only for gas, arriving at the motel just in time. We hadn't eaten, so we picked up sandwiches to go at a Denny's that was just closing, ate in the motel rooms, and collapsed. What a day!

A week later, we all went to Laughlin for a few days. We needed the R & R from our vacation. It had been the first vacation Fred had had in thirty years!

By now, Fred and I were making plans for our future together. We figured that by the following summer, Jon would want to be on his own, or with his girlfriend. He now had a car (well, buying it from Dad, using Dad's insurance, of course), a part-time job at Costco, had finally passed the driver's test, and, he said, enrolled in junior college. (He'd lied to Fred about taking classes the previous year.) We could, we decided, plan to m-m-m-marry (not easy for either of us to say!). Or, just live together? Nah, we couldn't! We knew that his family would be happy, and my family would be thrilled! My grandchildren were just waiting to call him Grandpa Fred, and my daughter and son-in-law would finally have a loving father.

At Christmas, we divided our time—presents, brunch, and playing games with my kids (Fred's a very competitive board game player); then dinner at his sister's, with Jon and his girlfriend. Things were looking great!

Fred got a call from his oldest girl, Cami, who had been diagnosed with autism as a child. However, she'd graduated high school and had been working full-time ever since she'd left her dad. Living with the two other girls (and, probably cleaning and babysitting for them), she had been brainwashed against her father. Now, she sobbed to Fred that she was in trouble, and the girls wouldn't let her stay with them anymore. She asked if she could come live with him. Fred heard the other girls, in the background, telling her what to say, and he smelled a rat. She stated that she'd been "naughty with a man," and they wanted her out. Fred knew better, but he tried to calm her down. He knew she couldn't live there with Jon, Jon's friend, Jerry, who was rooming with them, and the boys' girlfriends, who were often at the apartment, too. Fred was also afraid that it was some kind of a trap the girls had cooked up to hurt him, since he hadn't heard from any of them in five years. He knew Cami was scared, and told her he would call her the next day. Taking off work, he did some detective work. He found that one daughter wanted to live with an older woman, and the other's fiancé didn't want Cami living with them. So, they really were kicking her out! He called the girls' mother in Florida, and made arrangements for Cami to go there. Fred, though struggling with the decision to send her, figured that she'd at least be safe with her mom and step dad. She also had some money from the state for her disability, and she could easily find a job. And, no, Cami was not in trouble; she'd never even been out on a date! I had offered her a room at my place, but Fred felt that Cami was too afraid of him, let alone someone she didn't know. Picking her up at a designated spot, with her little bit of luggage, he drove her to Los Angeles Airport, stayed with her there, got permission to board with her, get her settled in her seat, and waited until the plane took off. Driving home, in tears, he'd lost his little girl, again. He was devastated!

Fred and I stayed home New Year's Eve, quietly enjoying each other, and toasting OUR NEW YEAR—2006! The next weekend, we were so tired and lazy, we just ate and napped. He felt that he had, somehow, strained a back muscle. With a promise to me that he would "see about it," when I asked him to make a doctor's appointment, he was about to head for home.

He said, "You know, we never even had our favorite form of entertainment!" I was shocked that we hadn't made love and begged him to stay a little longer, but he wouldn't.

I was making plans for Fred's fifty-fifth birthday, on January 30. At our singles meeting before his birthday, I surprised Fred with a decorated cake, candles, cards and balloons. The whole group sang to him. He was embarrassed, but happy and laughing.

"Oh, you just wait," he whispered. "I'll get you in April!"

I tried my damnedest to get him to come home with me that Tuesday night, but he just wouldn't. He said he had a big work day ahead, and tomorrow night, he, Jon, and Jon's friend, Jerry, were having a Boys' Night Out. So much for my feminine wiles!

Thursday morning, at 10:30, Jon called.

Oh, good, I thought, he's going to help me with Fred's birthday party.

"Hi, Jon."

"Joanne, Daddy's dead!" he sobbed.

"What?"

"Dad died last night . . . in his sleep."

> For, of all sad words
> Of tongue or pen,
> The saddest are these:
> "It might have been."

> —John Greenleaf Whittier, "Maud Muller"

Marie Thompson

Good storytellers have what I call "visual imagination."
That is, they are able to create or recreate people and places
for readers. Another great asset is originality, the ability to
give a new slant to the commonplace. In all my years of con-
ducting writing workshops for senior citizens (since 1997), I
have never encountered a more original writer than Marie
Thompson. Her images and figures of speech are strikingly
original (and apt)—for instance, "The cat stretched like
pulled taffy, yawing, exposing its lethal weapons." All of us
assumed her tale "The Button" was fact, but, in fact, it was
fiction. Of course, the unanswered question is intriguing:
Where did the idea for such a strange and wonderful tale
come from?

—W.R.W.

Another Chance

Dust particles played chase in the shafts of sunlight breaking through the windows. A large, tufted-ear marmalade cat lounged on the windowsill, eyes half closed as it watched the green budgerigar swinging on a perch in a white, elaborate pagoda. Colorful curtains hung from the two windows, freshly plumped cushions covered in the same fabric stood in line on the couch. The television was a monotone invasion, and entertained no one.

A tinkling of china cup against a saucer announced the occupant of this cozy, immaculate apartment. Florence was a large woman, wearing an overall emblazoned with roses of all colors. Her white sweater was slightly yellowed and matted through a multitude of washings. The pelmet of skirt below the cheerful overall was black, so too, were her stockings, covering thick, defiant legs. Her feet were enveloped in checkered brown slippers, a wobbling pompom atop each bobbed incessantly with each step. Her face was lined and set and she peered with dull eyes through rimless glasses. "Pretty boy!" she called to the bird, her voice frail, contrasting to her physical presence. She placed the cup of tea on the small table, and sat down in the large chair positioned purposely in the sunlight. The warmth penetrated her tired bones. Eventually, her body relaxed, melting into the fabric. She leaned her head back and felt at peace. Time passed slowly, the ticking of the clock competing with the television voices, companions for a lonely seventy-five year old widow.

Shadows grew into long, grotesque shapes across the room. The cat stretched like pulled taffy, yawning, exposing its lethal weapons. Florence stirred, her inner clock awakening her from the routine nap. Slowly, as her circulation improved, she arose, taking the teacup into the kitchenette. Five o'clock. Another day almost over. How endless they seemed. Stacked one upon the other, like the dishes in the cabinet on the wall in front of her; neat, uniform, one just like the other. The doorbell rang. Who could that be at this hour? She opened the door a couple of inches and saw an eager blond woman in her late 30's.

"Mrs. Walker, my name is Jackie Singleton. I'm a volunteer with the local support group for the elderly. Your name and address was given to me by your doctor's office, as you are within my area. I want to introduce you to our program. Can I come in for a minute? I know it's a bit late, but it's the first chance I've had all day." She insisted.

"Well, it is late, and I wasn't expecting company."

"I'll only take a moment. Really!"

Jackie sat herself in Florence's chair, ignoring the unwelcoming stare. She had several notes and proceeded to explain the program she ran. "Twice a week, Mondays and Wednesdays, we pick you up and take you to the senior center. You can mix with others, do crafts, read—do just about anything you want. It is a fun time, and will get you out a bit."

"I don't want to get out a bit."

"'Course you do. It will be good for you. You'll make friends and can even have lunch there. I'll pick you up on Monday, around ten. Be ready. I have to pick others up on the way." Jackie gathered up her purse and papers, extending a hand as she stood. Florence's hand felt lifeless, she gave it a gentle squeeze. "I'll let myself out, Mrs. Walker. I really hope you decide to join us. We'll come by, just in case. See you on Monday."

Fine rain had left a velvet sheen of droplets across the shoulders of Jackie's coat. The smell of wet wool was pungent, sweet. Icy wind had torched her nose and cheeks. The office offered no welcome; the furniture was sparse, leftovers gathered from who-knows-where. The electric fire was straining at impossible odds to overcome the damp, chilled air. She decided to keep her damp coat on, and turned her thoughts to Florence Walker. Family structure had changed drastically over the years. A place for a frail grandparent within the family unit was not the normal set-up any more. So many seniors, lonely, were just biding their time. Florence may be seventy-five, but she still had much to offer, and Jackie accepted the challenge of reawakening her. It was well past eight before all the reports had been written up. It had stopped raining, and abstract patterns of color from the streetlights reflected across the wet pavements. Jackie quickened her pace, glad to be going home at last.

Monday appeared bright, if not warm. The bare tree branches were black against a gray winter sky, while birds rested, feathers fluffed for warmth. The small white van was on time. To Jackie's pleasant surprise, so, too, was Florence, who felt a mixture of both excitement and fear. It had not been easy getting ready for the Center. Florence had sat on the edge of the bed, robe wrapped tightly around her, wondering what the day would bring. She later took care to dress well, choosing a blouse worn only once before, the pale blue bringing out the color of her eyes, softening the pallor of her face, but not its hard expression. She was afraid to soften, to feel. It cost too much. She placed a cameo broach framed in gold at the neckline, a gift from her husband, so long ago.

Jackie was hopeful as she buckled Florence into the van seat. They picked up five other passengers, eager, smiling—their steps hesitant against the weather. Jackie tenderly guided them into their seats.

The Center was a new red brick building tucked onto the end of a grand gothic church, and the disparity between old and new was striking. A tall, bespectacled man was waiting to greet them, cheery in his yellow sweater. His young companion, her chestnut curls dancing, helped him steer the flock into the warmth. She took Florence's arm as Florence slowly, insecurely, stepped along the path. "Thank you, dear." The girl smiled happily.

It took time to get everyone settled, but Florence just sat in a hard chair, refusing to participate in any craft or the sing-a-long, but Jackie allowed her to be. After a while, Florence found herself watching the young woman who had greeted her at the Center. There was something about her open smile, her eagerness to help, that touched Florence. Her laughter was childlike, innocent. Florence turned to the woman beside her who was working with deft fingers to create a table mat, her hands so thoroughly trained, concentration was unnecessary.

"That girl over there, the young one. Who is she?"

"That's Sue. She helps out here each week. Still lives at the orphanage although she's not a kid anymore; must be about eighteen. She earns her keep by doing odd jobs. She has a developmental disability, you know." Her words matter-of-fact, not unkind.

"What do you mean?"

"Can't speak properly, brain damaged. Don't think any family wanted her. She's a lovely girl though, always got a quick smile."

When lunch was wheeled into the dining area, Sue asked Florence if she was ready to take off her coat. Florence had purposely kept it on as her badge of defiance, wanting everyone to know she had little intention of staying. However, to her own surprise, she found it difficult to hold back from Sue. Florence slipped the coat from her shoulders, and emerged as if from a cocoon, in the pale blue dress with the broach at her throat. Jackie noticed the attention Florence had given to her appearance, and felt encouraged.

Florence went to the Center again on Wednesday, and watched Sue, taking in her dark, shining eyes, thick eyebrows and full mouth. Her curly hair bounced around her pale face, drawn for one so young. What was it that pulled her to the girl? Florence had her own children, four of them who lived busy, successful lives. They had no time for her beyond their duty performed by monthly checks. The grandchildren were growing into adults. She had missed their development, had not been included in their childhood antics, but kept as an outsider. What did their birthday cards mean to her when the warm words were backed by only cold indifference? "Time to go, Florence." Florence was surprised to see Jackie holding her coat. Where had the day gone?

As she turned the key in the lock, her spirits fell rapidly. Even the warmth of the cat curling around her ankles had no effect. Automatically, she turned on the television, needing to fill the noisy quiet. The apartment had always been her safe haven, so much a part of her, yet it suddenly became overbearing, pressing in. She embraced herself, needing to feel someone's arms around her, even if they were only her own. Tight sobs escaped her clamped lips and heavy tears broke from her eyes. She sat down in the armchair, unsteady.

Sue walked quickly. She wore a special boot that was hidden by her slacks. It had taken a lot of practice to not show a limp, and she was proud of her accomplishment. The wind blew hard, lifting and holding her long hair behind her, like a horse's mane, wild and free. She pushed her gloved hands deep inside her coat pockets and shivered. A gust of freezing air grabbed at her, grasped briefly before letting go with a shove, destabilizing her balance and composure.

Florence opened her front door, and stared in disbelief. A white, pinched face stared back, eyes wide, uncertain. "What are you doing here? What a lovely surprise."

Sue's mouth turned up in a grin of relief, teeth white against her chapped lips. She held out a small, crumpled envelope.

"Your broach."

Florence had missed it. Her long graceless fingers grasped Sue's arm and gently pulled her into the warm apartment.

"Let me make you a hot drink, you must be frozen. Take your coat off for a few moments and sit by the fire."

Sue made for the cat, picking it up by the front legs, the rest of its body hanging like unwound velvet. She pressed her nose against the warm softness, delighted her attention has been accepted. Florence brought in a steaming cup, the smell of chocolate strong and tempting.

"I appreciate you coming, Sue. How did you know the broach was mine?"

"Jackie told me to bring it to you. She gave me your address and told me how to get here." Her voice was out of tune, the words incomplete and rushed, as if needing to get out before forgotten.

Florence noticed Sue's sweater and slacks were worn, tight fitting hand-me-downs. A seam of the sweater was held together by large unmatched stitches. She assumed they were Sue's repair work. She smiled as Sue sipped noisily on the chocolate.

"Are you in a hurry? Can you stay a while?" Florence's voice was soft but prepared for rejection. "I can make us something to eat."

"If I'm not on time, they worry. I'll come again, though." Sue placed her empty cup down, reaching for her coat.

Florence watched from the window, as Sue hurried along the street, her figure bent against the wind. Suddenly she stopped, turned and waved—every part of her small body involved—then she was gone.

A fresh tablecloth covered the small table in front of the fire, and two chairs were placed across from each other. The firelight softened to elegance the small crystal vase containing plastic daffodils. A chocolate cake held place of honor, and crust-less sandwiches invited sampling. Almost one o'clock. Sue should be arriving any minute. Florence gently lifted the cat from her lap and peered through the window. Three months had past since she had first seen Sue at the Center. Three months of slow thawing. Feelings Florence had put on hold for so many years had begun to seep through her strong, built-to-last defenses. She had tried to hold back at the beginning, yet found herself looking forward to Mondays and Wednesdays, if only to see Sue. It had been a long time since she had looked forward to anything. Sue, too, looked forward to seeing Florence. As soon as the van drew up, Sue ran out to escort Florence, her small hand holding tightly onto Florence's arm.

The rhythm of the ticking clock became intense. It was now two-thirty, and still no Sue. What could have happened? Maybe she missed the bus, or perhaps she forgot. Florence's fingers absently worried a couple of crumbs on the cloth. By now the heat of the fire had dwindled. The chocolate frosting had softened and the sandwiches were drying out. She had taken pleasure in preparing the things Sue liked. Shadows stretched like misshapen fingers across the room. Florence cleared off the table as her anxiety increased.

The doorbell was shrill—the knocking urgent. Florence hurried to open the door, and peered into Sue's anxious eyes. "I missed the bus and had to walk. It was a long way." Her voice was stressed and reproachful. Florence drew her into her arms.

"I've been so worried," her voice breaking with relief. Florence reset the table while Sue took off her coat and reached for the cat.

"Jackie told me it's your birthday tomorrow. I've got you a present."

Sue's eyes sparkled with excitement. Florence felt childlike pleasure as she unwrapped the creased package. From the white tissue emerged bright pink satin slippers. "They're pretty. Those brown slippers you wear look like a grandpa's."

"You're quite right, dear, they are ugly old things. But these are beautiful!" Florence slipped her feet into the new slippers. She reached out and put her arms around Sue. They clung together. The emptiness they had both known for so long began to fill.

Over the next few weeks, they became inseparable, and Jackie helped Sue move in to Florence's spare room. One evening, Sue, fresh from the bathtub, sat on the arm of Florence's chair.

"Flo', I want to tell you about why I don't go to see anyone at the orphanage any more. I don't always understand things, and because of the way I talk, they get mad with me. They call me stupid, and that hurts my feelings. I don't have to go, do I, Flo?"

Florence felt anger rising. How blind some people could be, she thought, didn't they realize how much Sue had overcome?

"Of course not! You don't have to do anything you don't want to ever again. I've hurt, too. It started when my husband died. My children thought I hadn't cared, but I didn't know the seriousness of his illness. The doctor didn't know. There was a sudden rush to the hospital, and it was over so quickly."

"You mean your children get mad with you?"

"Yes. All three. Stephen lives only a few miles from here. He's named for his father. Joel is in New York, and Lisa's upstate. My husband and I were married for many years. We were very happy, always together." She smiled wistfully. "He was from Maine and sailed most of his life. I remember one summer when the kids learned to sail. He was so proud of them. They're blond like him—called them his little Vikings. That was a glorious vacation—we barbecued on the beach . . . rode our bikes. They grew like beanstalks that year, towering over me, just like their father." Florence looked far away. "I used to love to swim, and that's how we met. I was swimming in the bay and he went by in his dinghy, kept splashing me until I gave up and got on board. He was full of fun. He gave me the broach you found. I saw it in a jewelers shop window, and the next thing I knew, he had bought it for me. He was like that—so generous, so loving." She laughed, the happy memory softening her face to almost pretty. "I suppose it's hard for you to think of me as young *and* a swimmer. I was good at it, and won quite a few trophies. I taught my children." She paused and looked at Sue. "I could teach you. I'm not a youngster but still know how." She sighed quietly. "It all seems so long ago. I couldn't believe it when the doctor said it was all over. I seldom hear from my children now. They said I should have known their father was so ill, but I honestly didn't. No one did. Their accusations beat me down, turned me against myself. They moved away, one by one, as soon as they could. They pulled together, but left me an outsider. They never understood my heart was broken, too. There's talk from time to time about visiting, but they seldom make it. They're successful and send me money every month, but don't always remember my birthday, and at Christmas, I get a card with another check. I'd so like a visit, especially from my grandchildren. They're grown up now—but Joel's Ruth is still a teenager like you." Florence's voice was tense with emotion. "I've missed out on so much. My children had each other, but I had no one. I just closed up, kept my feelings to myself. I've been very lonely."

"You have me now, Flo', you don't have to be lonely any more. I remembered your birthday. I'll be your new granddaughter." She moved to Florence's lap, and put her head on her shoulder. "I was lonely, too. The other kids made fun of me because I couldn't keep up at school, so I got left behind. I knew some of the answers, but the words got mixed up. The kids called me bad names and that made me cry. They said my mother and father didn't want me because I was stupid."

Florence stroked Sue's damp hair. "Jackie said they were very young and couldn't keep you. It must have been very, very hard for them to give you up. I'm certain your mother and father loved you. You know I do! You will always be a part of them and, of course, they are a part of you. They would be thrilled to see what a beautiful young girl you are." She smiled.

"You think I'm beautiful, Flo'? When ladies and men came to see the kids, they never wanted to see me. Then I got older so I knew I wouldn't get adopted, ever."

"If I'd known you then, I'd have adopted you." Florence hugged Sue to her. "Don't be sad any longer—we've found each other now, and yes, you will be my new granddaughter." Sue pressed herself against Florence—her small body fitting perfectly in Florence's arms.

"Shall I call you Grandmother?"

"If you like. Flo's all right, though."

"I think I'll choose . . ." she put her finger to her lip and giggled with delight. "Umm . . . Grandmother!"

"That's settled then!"

There was no pity as each told their stories, and the words gushed out, cleansing. Exhausted, yet refreshed from sharing, Sue and Florence smiled at each other. They knew the past was over and they had a chance for a new beginning. Sue settled herself in front of the fire, with the cat on her lap. Florence went into the kitchen to make hot milk

"How did you get into the Senior Center?" Flo called.

"Oh, because I'm older, I had to get a job. Not in a shop or anything 'cos that would be too hard for me. Jackie used to work with adoptions at the orphanage and saw me one day, and asked if I'd like to help her. She said she needed someone at the Center, someone who could make tea and greet the visitors, and things like that. I said I wanted to work."

"Well, you do a great job there! I don't know what we'd do without you!"

"Flo', I mean Grandmother, I still earn some money, I can give to you!" Sue's eyes were shining.

"My dear, I've got more than enough of my own. That's yours. In fact, we can go shopping tomorrow." She put the tray down on the table by the chair and handed Sue a cup of warm milk. "It'll be fun! You can buy something you really like."

It was a warm spring day. Crocuses would soon be pushing through the hard soil, and eventually bluebells would carpet the woods. It was a time of anticipation and hope. Florence was at the front of the Center. Her smile was cheerful as she stepped forward to welcome the van when it drove up. "Come along, everyone, I've fresh coffee made. Hello, John, glad you could make it today. You look much better. Sue, give Mrs. Jason a hand with her bag, will you?"

Florence took delight in playing the role of mother hen. The Center had developed into a social club—a noisy metropolis of activity, rather than just a place to go to fill in time. The members had become close-knit, watchful for each other. Sue had involved a few friends from an assisted living facility over the last few weeks and they, too, had become a part of this unique community. Some had trouble keeping arms and legs from jerking like puppet limbs, while others spoke with difficulty or were unable to take direction easily. No matter. A partnership was formed through love and tolerance. No longer labeled handicapped, disabled or old, they were just people, coming together and enriched by the experience. Florence's involvement with Sue had enabled her to rediscover herself, and she had been completely accepted by the Center. No matter what her mood, a smile and warm encouragement always greeted her. Florence put her arm around Sue's shoulders as they made their way into the building, stopping occasionally to exchange a word with a member or two. Anyone passing by could hear the spontaneous, delighted laughter, and perhaps would recognize the devotion between grandmother and granddaughter walking off in the distance.

The Norton Simon

Walking around the galleries of an art museum is a treat beyond description for me. I often travel the 605 and 210 freeways to the Norton Simon in Pasadena. I like its size—not as large and busy as galleries in Los Angeles—and the patrons who meander along with me are patient and polite if one wants—needs, to stay awhile with a particular piece of artwork. The museum was renovated a few years ago and now includes small rooms off the main galleries. I like the design because one can spend time in an intimate space that is virtually silent. It allows a solitary experience—just you and the artwork. The silence offers one the luxury of study, a close-up that exposes brush strokes, texture and the depth of the palette used. I feel the intensity of the powerful life-size Rodin figures that are set upon the grassy knolls along the walkway to the entrance. Their strength, their weight, contrast with the delights of the light and colors of the Impressionists' work that line the walls of the large open space of the main gallery. Cézanne's *Tulips in a Vase* is the commissionaire welcoming the visitor through the entrance doors.

In the first gallery, just to the right, is a small room with walls lined in red silk. Displayed on the right hand wall, surrounded by small pastoral scenes, is one of my favorite paintings. It is not one that catches the eye easily as the colors are subtle, restful. But it calls to me. It is Jean-Desire-Gustave Courbet's seascape *Marine,* painted in 1865–66. A little over 19" x 24", the picture is composed of bands of pale pinks and yellows, and hinges on the abstract. No boat or other typical ocean element is included. The sandy shore is covered in blue and gray tide pools that reflect a blustery autumn sky. No figure explores these craters, perhaps filled with tiny creatures trapped for a limited time by an ebbed tide. Courbet used a palette knife to agitate the surface paint, exposing the lighter shades below. It is without harsh lines, just a blending of color that draws me in towards the last remnants of a rosy sunset. The desolation brings a chill to my skin, yet I stay.

Further on, towards the end of the main gallery are several other works by Courbet. They are so varied in subject as well as technique, one questions if they are works by the same artist. His gentle landscapes with waterfalls and fauna can be compared to Gainsborough, but his boats resting on sandy shores or navigating vicious rocks are unquestionably his own. His portraits express lively energy through color, and light in a focused eye holds the viewer for an extra moment.

Two pieces of sculpture have captured me: Degas' *Little Dancer Aged Fourteen*, is a 38" high wax figure of a girl dressed in a real silk bodice and gauze tutu, wrinkled tights and ballet slippers. She even wears a satin ribbon through her wig of real hair. The figure is completely covered with a fine layer of wax to unify the image while revealing the texture of each piece of fabric. The late nineteenth century public expressed mixed reactions to this arresting figure, but my own response has always been utter delight.

The other piece I make sure I spend time with is Marino Marini's abstract bronze, *Horseman*. When I look upon this 40" high image, I cannot help smiling. The plump Horseman is firmly seated on the ample rump of a horse that calmly gazes down over its left leg—at what, one can imagine. The rider appears exuberant, his head is tilted upwards towards the sky, while his hands rest gently onto the animal's back. To me, this sculpture represents wonder about life and is a celebration of just that. The simplistic style ensures nothing interferes with the peaceful, blissful energy I feel each time I visit.

The lovely Tranquil Garden, complete with a large pond where dragonflies hover, and specimen trees blend to a restful panorama, is a respite for aching feet and an overworked eye. A cup of coffee restores energy so one can continue the stroll through a wonderland. Conversations go on around me, but I am oblivious because my concentration is on the remarkable pieces that remain in my mind's eye, and those that are yet ahead of me. Happily, if my energy level doesn't recover, I know I can return again. And again.

The Scruff

There is a small stray cat that roams our street block like a homeless waif who looks upon the world with eyes that challenge, dare. I'm convinced he is a male because there is no way a feminine gene could exist within that feisty, moth-eaten character. He wanders the gutters, often full of dried leaves and water run-off, and spends lazy hours basking in the sun, head propped up against the curb, eyes not quite closed, so a thin line of pale yellow affirms he is ever vigilant and in control. I know people who place themselves in a similar position, but spread out on a chaise lounge. When I take my daily walks, he stares across the road at me, but makes no move. Those yellow eyes are emotionless, as if cataracts of dust cloud over them, distorting his view of the world by extracting interest in life beyond his chosen territory. He reminds me of a shapeless rag rug, the kind made from patches of material taken from old clothing. My grandmother made one from my brother's gray school uniform trousers, and it was placed inside her front door to wipe our feet on before continuing down the hall. It was anything but pretentious but served its purpose extremely well for years. This cat is remarkably similar—a well-used patchwork of black, gray and ginger—the colors now faded by dirt and burrs.

Although tangles and fur clumps prevent a full stride, he ambles along very well, increasing the lackadaisical saunter to an impressive pace when necessary. My neighbor directly across from me feeds the strays from the area twice a day, and this errant spirit meanders to her front porch with a swagger that is impressive enough to ensure other hungry drifters take the second seating. The menu is unchanging: Friskies, on time and plentiful. Around sunup, a damp shadow slinks along the side of the road. Is it too hungry or could it be too stubborn to avoid a shower from the early morning sprinklers in order to eat first? As daylight increases, the shadow turns out to be the street tough. He emerges from the porch to survey those subservient felines, waiting patiently for their own breakfast; they know their place. He takes his time, as if acknowledging his power to prolong their hunger pangs. Once his own appetite is satiated, he parks himself on the raised doorstep. Leisurely licking his paws, he acts out a charade of grooming and, with a gray tongue, cleans off a last crumb from those tight, thin lips. His ablutions completed, he nonchalantly strolls away, looking back once, as if to say, okay boys, now go and get it. At six-thirty precisely in the evening, he returns for dinner, and the whole show starts over again. Did T.S. Eliot have such a character in mind for his book of poems *Old Possums Book of Practical Cats?* But, then, Old Deuteronomy was too much the groomed gentleman in Andrew Lloyd Webber's adaptation for his Broadway show, *CATS*.

I was taking the trashcans in from the curb a couple of days ago. Dusk was just settling in, the remaining light beginning to fade like a soft breath. Wafts of star jasmine perfume filled the cooling air. Kitchen windows of the single story stuccos glowed invitingly as evening meals were being prepared. In the middle of the road sat our boy intently cleaning himself. This was an unusual sight, and I wished I had a camera handy— a photograph would be proof. He looked worse than usual. He must have rolled in grass cuttings, for green spikes were sticking out all over him like bobby pins trying to tame a wacky hairstyle. With one leg straight up against his shoulder, he was attending to his belly. Upon seeing me, he paused, stared coldly as if saying, *got something on your mind?* Through telepathy, I replied, *I'm not getting into it with you,* and turned my back.

Later, when I took my dog for her evening stroll, a passing car swerved, its headlamp beaming over the body of a small animal lying flat on the asphalt of the road. I could see a patch of moisture under it, and there was no movement. My breath caught in my throat. Oh, no! The beastie has been run over! Telling my dog to stay on the sidewalk, I went over to the motionless bundle and bent down, slowly putting my hand out and calling softly. No response. I stepped closer. He abruptly lifted his head and two menacing amber bolts of light stared back at me. The unexpected movement startled me, causing me to lose my balance and I fell over on my side. The asphalt was still warm from the day's heat, and I realized this was what *that* rogue was taking advantage of. He stretched up and came to stand close to my face. Head down, he snarled, baring his teeth. HIISSSSS! The fetid stink of cesspit living rose up. I watched as he turned and unhurriedly walked across to the other side of the street. We have a

Neighborhood Watch for such a person, but what can you do about a cat? I smiled, and thought, not without pride, *that's my boy!*

The Button

I'd been walking for about a couple of miles—the ocean was in a calm mood, and gently lapped against the shore, leaving a delicate lace of bubbles. I was not the only intruder that early hour; the wet sand was already agitated by legions of footprints. Surfers, waiting patiently for a wave that would provide the addictive thrill, were like a pod of porpoise. Their wetsuit uniforms neutered any individuality. Groups of gray and white plovers raced to the water's edge. Bills at the ready, they speared a tasty morsel with precise timing, and then as a single body, abruptly sped to dry safety. Their focus was unwavering as I walked beside them. I picked up a small, fan-shaped shell, and rinsed it in the cool water. I had quite an assortment in my plastic sandwich bag by now, enough to cover a picture frame I intended as a gift for a friend. I turned and started back, walking slowly, resisting. The sand was beginning to absorb the heat from the sun, and I puckered my toes in delight. Straggly lengths of dried seaweed and odd shapes of driftwood added to the litter scattered by unthinking intruders—plastic bottles, pieces of balloons—even a sandal. I collected as I walked, and quickly my arms were full. Frustrated, I dumped the junk into a trash bin.

"Terrible, isn't it?" I looked over. A young man was waxing a surfboard.

"It is! Makes me really mad." Something caught my eye. I bent to pick it up.

"What ya' got there?"

"It's a button—a brass button." I held it out and he came over.

"Never seen anything like that before. Seems out of place here."

I rubbed the sand off, and saw the embossed shape of a five-petal flower. I turned the button over in my hand. The sand had worked the metal so it was polished and bright. I slipped it into my pocket, and walked on.

Upon arriving at my home, I took the bag of shells out to the patio to rinse off residue with the garden hose. Placed together on the table, the shells looked pale, anemic, but the spray brought out a bright palette of orange, blues, browns and cream, brilliance usually revealed to only those who patrol beneath the waves. Quickly, the heat of the sun returned the colors to subtle opaque. It was peaceful in the garden, and I lost myself in the pleasure of coating a picture frame with porcelain-like fans, no less delicate than those fluttered by graceful geishas.

Pleased with my finished creation, I wandered into the bathroom to clean up. My pockets were sticky with salt and sand, and I stripped carefully. I'd learned sweeping up those tiny granules was a thankless job, and was still challenged to get rid of those that seemed to procreate in the corners of the baseboard. I found the brass button in my pant pocket, and placed it in the soap dish.

It was a few days later before I took up the button again. It had been so out of place on the sand. Did it wash up from a land far, far away—carried on the heavy curves of undulating swells, racing toward a final destination, or was it simply tossed away because the trashcan was inconveniently out of reach? I pressed my thumb against the embossed flower and absently put it back into the soap dish where it remained for several weeks, building up a coating of soap deposits and tarnish. I got so used to it being there, I didn't notice it any more. It was quite some time later before we got reacquainted. Friends were coming over, and the house got a thorough cleaning to save my reputation. I scrubbed the hardened crust of soap and was pleased to see the brass polish up quite nicely. The back of the button showed small chips and an indentation as if its journey to the California shore had been a rough one. It was only about an inch across and was void of any number or word. Where had it come from? Whose hand had crafted its manufacture? I took it into my office and placed it on my desk. Friends would soon be arriving for dinner, and I still had a couple of things to prepare in the kitchen.

I had a number of letters to write and decided on a wet spring morning to show some discipline, and tackle at least a couple. Once I got going, it was easy to lose myself in internal dialogue through written words. I felt close to my father so many miles away in England as I told him about new seeds I'd planted in the garden, how the southern California sandy soil took a lot of replenishing to bring about my desired display of color and variety, and what plants I had chosen to encourage birds and friendly insects. I complained about the hardship of getting lupine seeds to germinate in the coastal climate. His garden was a mass of purple and pink spikes, coming up year after year without any codling. My obedience to friendly suggestions had resulted in plants two to three inches tall; then, for some mysterious reason, they shriveled and died. I told him I was not about to give up, however, and had already sowed a row of seeds softened by a thirty-six hour soaking in an effort to encourage their sprouting. I signed my name at the bottom of the page and felt acutely aware of the miles separating us. I addressed the envelope and, as it was my practice to display my bragger individuality, placed a thick blob of black wax on the back flap. It was then that the button caught my eye and, almost absently, I picked it up and pressed it against the soft warm wax. The imprint of the flower was perfect, and complimented the subject of my screed to my father. I happily mailed the letter later that day.

I continued to use the button when sealing personal correspondence, and even had a block made so I could add it to my signature or stamp a piece of stationery. That little flower became my trademark. It became so well known to family and friends that it was unnecessary for my name to appear in order to be identified. In a burst of creative energy, I copied the design and made brooches from tiny smooth cockleshells gathered from the sands at low tide. I glued five individual pieces in place onto a metal clip, and then added a coat of varnish to bring out the colors of calcium build up. Nature had produced a subtle work of art, and it was satisfying to see friends wearing these little badges of alliance.

It was probably about a year later when I had lunch with a couple of British friends. We were to discuss the possibility of becoming U.S. citizens. They had brought along a middle-aged Asian woman who was giving consideration to the same idea. May Kuboto was Japanese, and had been living in California with her family for twenty years. Her short straight hair was tinged with silver, but her skin was as smooth as silk. She must have been in her sixties and, perhaps because of the fat-rich diet of this wealthy society, was as rounded as a melon. She had a gentleness and grace about her, and I found myself immediately drawn to her. At the end of two very pleasant hours, we stood outside the restaurant to say our goodbyes. May hesitated for a moment, and then pointed to the shell pins we were wearing, and asked about their significance. I explained about finding the brass button and its influence in the pin creation, and resolved to give her one next time we got together.

May came to tea a couple of weeks later, and it was fun to discuss the differences and similarities of our particular cultures when it came to tea ceremonies. I'd set up a tray complete with a fine starched cotton cloth, my porcelain china, a selection of finger sandwiches and petit fours, and placed it on a small table in front of where I would sit. My teapot was large, and covered in a quilted *cozy* to keep the contents hot. My cups were large. Even the plates seemed large, although they were the smallest of the set. As May draped a napkin across her lap, and helped herself to a sandwich, I could see the difficulty she was having in balancing a cup of hot tea in one hand and a plate on her knee. As May explained, the Japanese serve their tea in very small cups from very small pots, and are usually seated in front of a low table on which to place the china. There is no milk or sugar involved as with the British brew—just refreshing understated tasting tea. The British ritual seems awkward in comparison and certainly required skills I hadn't contemplated before. Perhaps our larger Western legs provided a wider surface for plate balancing as we sipped. We were soon laughing at such antics and quickly moved ourselves to a more comfortable spot at the dining table. May proudly explained that in Japan, the tea ceremony is a traditional ritual influenced by Zen Buddhism; water represents *yin* and the fire used to heat the water is *yang*. Even modern Japanese practice Tea as an important social event from which they feel a sense of national belonging. Harmony is sought with the environment and all others through concentration on beautiful rituals, self-discipline and personal discovery. Sharing a cup of tea with family and friends was an immensely important and pleasurable time out for both of us, a respite if you will. May's voice was soft and wistful, and I became aware of my own intense homesickness.

It was on May's third visit when I gave her a shell pin, welcoming her to our small fraternity. Her almond shaped eyes glistened with pleasure. On impulse, I got the brass button from my office to show her the impetus behind its design. She took the button and gazed at it in silence for a moment or two.

"It's Japanese," she said.

I was dumbfounded. "I've wondered where it came from. I found it on the beach over a year ago."

"It's a naval uniform button from the Second World War."

"Are you sure? You can tell just like that?"

"My father was an officer in the Japanese Imperial Navy. He was killed in 1943, so I don't remember him, but my mother kept his dress uniform on display. Buttons like this one were on his jacket. As a little girl, I would help my mother polish them with brass cleaner. I think she held on to the hope if she kept the uniform impeccable, it would somehow bring him back. It took years for her to admit he would not return."

"Those were terrible years for so many." I put my hand on May's arm. "I'm glad we're friends."

May squeezed my hand. "Yes, me, too."

I sat for a long time after May left. I absently rubbed the button against my thumb and thought of the journey this small fastener had taken. Had it been on the uniform of a proud officer killed in action, or just fallen from a slack thread due to slovenliness? How many storms and currents had it taken to land it on Sunset Beach, California? How had it avoided being swallowed by a hungry deep-water shadow? Or had it? Questions and more questions. I found myself smiling. This small, insignificant object had come thousands of perilous miles over a period of many decades, to eventually rest in the hand of a British immigrant walking along a Californian beach on a spring morning. It seemed ironic that a floral motif—seemingly so without malice, so mundane—identified an enemy naval officer and now, so many years later, had become my logo of recognition. I thought of all who had fought in a war where butchery took place beside heroics; those men and women draped in khaki, navy or air corps blue, sons and daughters, husbands and wives marched into hell while the band played on. Well, this small object had brought about a friendship that transcended all of that. On my next visit to May's immaculate and peaceful apartment, I gave her the button in a small dark blue leather box. After all, it belonged to her. We are U.S. citizens now, but May has a special kinship, because these California shores gave her father back to her—all because of a small, sand-polished, brass button.

An Enchanted Oasis

This past week I watched a brown pelican with its six foot wingspan circle a lake several times, until possibly the temptation of cool water became too much. Positioning itself for landing, its large head rested back against sturdy shoulders, it made a final turn. With large yellow webs stretched wide, it skied to a smooth stop and folded up those giant wings. The resulting wake unsettled the water, but not those swimming close by. Each went about its own business, seemingly more important than this visitor. In spite of water thick with silt and flotillas of food wrappings, a female mallard with metallic blue wing flashes, took newly hatched chicks for a swim, her muted brown feathers a soft place for one or two to hitch a ride. Light bathed the iridescent green of the male's head as he performed his fatherly duties as a distant sentinel.

You know that feeling when your eye takes in so much beauty, you forget to breathe? That's my experience each time I go to this park near my home. It's a small oasis that offers time out from pastel stucco and traffic emissions. About five acres, it includes a small island in a moat of murky water, and is a perfect habitat for waterfowl. When cool grass meets my sticky feet, I stretch my toes in delight and seem weightless, free. Heavy leafed willow, maple, and eucalyptus bounce in ocean breezes, producing a rustling that sounds to me like Nature's music.

There was a time when I passed by, driving without a second glance, my mind too busy to notice what was being offered. Then, on an impulse one hot afternoon, I parked on the roadside, took my sandals off, and entered a pocket of timelessness. My cluttered thoughts calmed and my spirit elevated as I allowed the tranquility to take over. The ducks and birds were just a part of the scene at first, but, over time, I became aware of not only the beauty of each species, but also the uniqueness of each individual. I was surprised when I recognized I'd become a bird watcher or, more precisely, a waterfowl watcher. With identity book and binoculars at the ready, I've learned to identify shapes, colors and group behaviors, and my eye can now distinguish the subtle differences. Each visit brings enchantment and discovery.

I've returned to this magical place many times, and now readily distinguish individuals with characteristics I've personified. A plump Ross goose has a damaged left wing so its flight feathers stand perpendicular—I've made him the designated greeter. Small groups of black-necked Canada geese ransacking the banks for prime greens, look comical with grass stuck to their glossy bills, and seem puzzled at my laughter. There's the blue heron, a dutiful sentry standing silently in the under-growth of the island. He is totally still as he con-templates the antics of half a dozen white-billed coots, their heads pumping back and forth to promote their progress across the lake, greenish webbed feet churning debris of leaves, bread and plastic. White geese with yoke-yellow bills honking their authority, assemble in the distance, water droplets scattered over their feathers sparkle in the sunlight.

I sometimes forget this remarkable place is not my personal property—certainly a sense of ownership came early, and when occasionally high, excited voices from the children's playground in the distance break into my consciousness, I'm startled. Not for long, how-ever, because I have a show to watch. My focus is on the two Brandt's cormorants poised in the eucalyptus to my right, and there, over on the island, several white egrets balance on the tops of swaying oak trees.

Recently, a small truck pulled up at the curb and an elderly man got out hauling a bag of seed. A quick eye and a piercing honk is all it took to create the ensuing frenzied feeding. I watched. The man was surrounded by a pool of turbulence. He called out to me, wanting—needing—to share his delight.

"Come here as often as I can, you know."

"Yes, I know."

No more needed to be said.

Sanctuary

I needed to buy a new armchair. Coming to the decision was not so difficult. The raspberry-pink velvet chair in my bedroom had faded badly. I thought it beautiful when new, but it's next to the sliding doors leading to the garden and gets a direct hit down the right side from the afternoon sunlight. I like this chair. It has a wide seat so that a cushion could be squeezed either side of me whenever I snuggled down in it to read a book or just to stare into space. It is that type of chair—one you can just lose yourself in. I've had it for years—twenty, at least. It has a history: this is where I nursed my babies, where I discovered the length of their eye lashes, the gentle arch of their brows, and where they metamorphosed from small, helpless bundles to chubby, responsive beings. There were never complaints when piles of clothing were dumped all over it, because I was too lazy to fold and put them away. Visitors have sat uncomfortably when their sense of duty brought them to me during my bout with cancer. It embraced me when the first clump of my hair fell out onto the book I was reading, and held on tight when the tears fell. When I was feeling weak and nauseated, it was like sitting in a friend's arms—you know, hugged, supported while I grew stronger. It's been a good chair—a partner, actually.

I've scouted a few department stores, sitting in woven rattan, wooden rockers, and upholstered high backed designs, but, somehow, none quite fitted me. I tried—really. I placed my arms on their straight arms, let my hands relax in my lap, and jiggled my seat to fit into the contour of their seats, but I didn't get that sense of coziness I was looking for. I then explored designer boutiques where there was an abundance of very opulent overstuffed chairs and a selection of beautiful fabrics, so many, I was rendered impotent to choose. I will confess it was fun to pretend I could afford a couple of the raw silks or brocades, and I enjoyed the assistant's help in directing me towards contrasts and trims. I was at the point of almost giving in because the persuasion was skillful but quite subtle. A rich cream taffeta caught my eye. I actually could see the chair in my room. Although it was too large, and I would need to compress every inch of me to get passed to the armoire, it certainly looked good with its gold braided trim. Very good indeed. Fortunately, I came to my senses before signing a contract that would have led to bankruptcy.

I arrived home deflated in spirit but not defeated. I wandered into my bedroom and unconsciously sat in the seat that had the lasting dip of my bottom, the imprint of my back—I fitted in perfectly. The new chairs I'd sat in had held an impression of me, but only for a fleeting moment, not permanent, like this old friend. I

curled up, and leaned my head back, my fingers absent-
ly rubbing the worn, thin areas along the arms. The
garden was growing quiet in the fading light. Starlings
and house sparrows gathered a last meal before settling
in for the night. The big marmalade tomcat from next
door, gliding along the wall, his head down and tail up
in a soft curl, showed little interest in their activity. He
was on his way to his own feast lovingly dished out by
his elderly owner, Mrs. Potter. I settled in the warmth
of the faded velvet. It wasn't long before I found my-
self fighting my eyelids to stay open, but I nodded off,
and awoke to cosseting darkness. I got up and switched
on the lamp. There was no more garden to look at,
but a reflection of me and my friend looking peaceful
together in a room that is cozy and complete. I smile
because a realization had occurred. This chair must re-
main—it has earned that right. It's a chronicle of fam-
ily events. I can look at a soft stain and tell you exactly
how it came about and who made it. I traced the faint
splotches where I'd tried to sponge off ink where my
daughter had practiced her letters. It was impossible for
her to keep the pen from overlapping the paper. That
was when she was five—fifteen years ago. A friend, a
true friend, isn't discarded just because it's gained a few
rough patches and a worn skin. The bald patches in the
places where my body has rested is a body-print of me.

We have a connection, this chair and me. I no lon-
ger feel embarrassed by its worn, misshapen bulk, only
pride and gratitude. I continue to sit inside its peaceful
arms, listen to the rain, hug a new grandchild, or read
a book. You see, it is where I belong. This is my haven,
my place—my sanctuary.

Phan Vũ

Phan Vũ has this to say about his life: "I became aware of the imminent dangers to my life, my family, and my country, in my early adolescence when I saw the Japanese overthrow the French rule in Vietnam, capture Frenchmen and drive them along a street in Qui Nhơn City. Later, the raging Vietnam War dominated my adult life, directing my activities; either happy moments, or painful ones. At last, at the age of 60, I became completely free: beginning a new life, a free life, in a new country—the United States, with a new citizenship—American; and learning a new language—English."

Phan's contribution to our workshop was a historical novel, set in Viet Nam during and just after the infamous war. For a variety of reasons, we greatly enjoyed this writing. It is a touching love story, but it is also a rich portrait of a culture: landscapes, foods, social customs, economy.

With Phan's work, the question of language arose. Should he have someone regularize his language (i.e., edit it to meet the various strictures of what we call edited standard English), or should he retain the slight tinge of English-as-a-second-language that characterized his writing? The consensus was that he should retain the slightly "foreign" nature of his prose, for, after all, he was "translating" Vietnamese into English. His style added to the effectiveness of his story.

In the following selection, one finds both his slightly exotic (and effective) style and his rich portrayal of life in his native land.

—*W.R.W.*

Autumn Love

Following a long ride, sitting as a passenger on a wooden seat in a horse-drawn cart, Phương felt very uncomfortable. The red soil road the cart was riding on had many big and small potholes. The cart shook every time it slumped into one, or dipped into a rut. When his body hit the steel side of the cart, it hurt him. He also bent his head to avoid bumping into the sheet metal top. He had been reluctant to take this journey because his mother's health was too fragile to endure a 300-mile-long trip. But it had been a long time since his uncle left the family and devoted himself to a religious life in a remote countryside. Therefore, his mother wanted him to get to know his uncle, and to report how her brother was doing.

The cart traveled through several villages and in front of small rustic brick houses built along the road. Each dwelling had a garden of banana and jackfruit trees. Two old men, sitting on stools, playing chess beside a teapot and two cups, took a quick look at the passing cart, and then stared back at their game. A young woman carried a cluster of green and yellow bananas, followed by a small kid. Near naked, he wore only black shorts. The child was smiling and waving to the cart. Unlike Saigon, life was very quiet here.

The cart stopped at a pathway. The driver pointed to a small winding trail and said, "Young man, get off here and follow that trail, it leads to the pagoda on the top of the hill."

"Thank you, and here's the fare," Phương replied.

"Have a good day and take care."

"You, too, *Uncle*."

Alighting from the cart, Phương carried a gripsack in one hand and a bag in the other. The trail was steep and slippery because of yesterday's rain. Halfway up, he sat down for a rest on a big flat stone. As soon as he was going to climb up again, a novice Buddhist monk smiled at him.

"Are you going to the pagoda to say prayers?" he asked.

Phương did not say a word. He was stunned by the novice's smiling mouth, and by his beautiful eyes. He thought, how nice he is, and how soft and clear his voice sounds. The novice was waiting for Phương's answer.

"Oh, no . . . and yes," he replied. The novice laughed at Phương's funny reply.

"Yes, I want to spend some time in the pagoda to learn Buddha's teachings," Phương said. "And no, the Venerable is my mother's brother. I would like to see him because my mother worries about his health."

"I see. So, you're the Master's nephew, aren't you?" The novice concluded, with a smile.

Right away, Phương was attracted to this novice and he had a strong sympathy for him. Reaching the yard gate of the pagoda, the novice stopped and waited for Phương.

"How do you feel now? Tired or what?"

"Not much. Fresh air makes me fine."

"What's your name, sir?" The novice asked.

"Please call me Phương. What's yours?"

"I go by Vạn Lộc," said the novice. "How long are you going to stay with the Master?"

"From ten days to two weeks."

Now Phương had time to examine the novice. He was about 17 or 18. He wore long dark brown clothes, a brown cap, and black sandals.

"I will take you to the parlor and let the Venerable know of your arrival," Vạn Lộc said. He then left.

Phương set the bag on the table and took out two robes, one brown and one gray, and two sweaters. Then he sat down on a wooden chair. The furniture was simple and made of wood and rattan. On the walls, there were pictures of Buddha, and other saints he did not know of.

The Venerable appeared at the door, followed by Vạn Lộc.

"Hello there, Phương. How're you doing? How's your mom?"

"Good afternoon, Uncle. Mummy's fine."

Vạn Lộc laughed and said, "Please call the Venerable, *Master*. He's Buddha's man, now."

"Oh, I am sorry," Phương smiled, looking at him. "I'm fine. It's been a long time since mom didn't heard any news from you, Master. She's a little bit worried about your health. So she sent me here to bring you some clothes."

"Now, you see me," the Venerable said. "Report to your mom how I am and tell her not to worry about my health. When I was young, your mother took good care of me. Now I am old, she still cares about me. She's a very good sister. Tell me about yourself."

"I'm a senior student at Saigon Law School. I'm taking a summer vacation."

"Okay. Stay here as long as you wish. Enjoy the vegetarian food and this peaceful hill site with fresh air. Vạn Lộc, take him to the guest room and see to what's needed."

"Yes, Master," Vạn Lộc answered.

Vạn Lộc showed Phương his room and its bathroom. The room had a bamboo bed with two blankets, a pillow and a mosquito net. A commode and a table were set beside the window. In the bathroom, a faucet supplied piped water to a big earthenware jar full of water.

"Oh—running water!" Phương shouted, surprised.

"I set up this water system two years ago," Vạn Lộc said.

At six p.m., Vạn Lộc told Phương to have dinner in the dining room. Phương was informed that the Master had had dinner before them. Phương was introduced to the cook and two other novices. The cook was a skinny old man. His speech was slow, and his attitude, polite. Inviting Phương to take a seat, he said that he was not a good cook. However, he had tried his best to make it appetizing for Phương. The two novices were about twenty years older than Vạn Lộc, and looked rather healthy and strong. Although there was no meat or fish, Phương ate well because the taste was new to him. The meal was basically fried soybean curd, roasted peanuts, vegetables, and fragrant rice. During the meal, they talked less, maybe due to reticence or shyness.

After dinner, Phương came back to his room. He went to bed, and right away slept like a stone. He had been told that he would not have to get up for the Morning Prayer. The morning meal would be served at about eight a.m. There would be a light lunch with fruit or sweet soup. So he could sleep as long as he liked.

In the morning, after a long, good sleep, Phương felt terrific. He came down to the dining room to have breakfast. Vạn Lộc greeted him with a big smile. Something charming on Vạn Lộc's face pleased Phương very much.

"Hi. How're you doing this morning, Phương?" The novice asked.

"I feel wonderful. How are you, Vạn Lộc?" Phuong replied.

"Fine, thanks. Did you sleep well last night?"

"I woke up only when you knocked on the door."

"Today I will take you for a sightseeing tour around the pagoda and the area surrounding the hills," the novice said.

"That sounds interesting," Phương replied.

"Make sure you have a big breakfast. We won't have lunch. We take only two handfuls of glutinous rice cooked with black beans and two bottles of water."

"Don't worry. I can spend all day without eating."

"And you don't drink water all day, do you?" Vạn Lộc inquired.

"Yes, I have to."

Both laughed cheerfully. Then they set off with their bamboo backpacks on their backs. They came to the main building consisting of a large hall perfumed with a fragrant scent. A majestic golden statue of Buddha sat on a shining teakwood altar placed against the brownish yellow wall of the hall. Large dishes of different-colored fruits and vases of varied flowers were among burning candles set on bright-bronze candlesticks and bowls of joss sticks, each spiraling out smoke that scented the room with a sweet smell. Before the altar stood a table, on which there was a wooden tocsin (bell) and a small black bronze bell for the Venerable to say prayers. The floor was covered with large colorful sedge mats. The main building faced the East to the Pacific Ocean. Then Phương and the novice stepped out into the solid red-tile bell shack. The black bell was about two feet in diameter and three feet high. A six-inch by eight-inch wood striker was hung on a beam.

Vạn Lộc said, "The bell clangs very far. The echoes of its sounds during the morning prayers awake farmers and workers living in the surrounding villages. The same echoes in the evening call them back home."

On the park surrounding the main house, big trees with large foliage gave cool shade to Buddhist believers and their children gathering for holiday celebrations. Adjacent to the main building were two long dwellings composed of rooms for guests, novices and the cook. Vạn Lộc's and Phương's rooms were in the southern residence; the dining room, the kitchen, and the storage, in the western house.

Vạn Lộc took Phương to the brook that had been harnessed to irrigate the fields and provide the pagoda with water. Vạn Lộc said, "Its flow is stronger in the rainy season than in the dry season. Two years ago, I asked the Master for permission to build this cement tank. As this stream is higher than the level of the pagoda complex, water runs to pipes in every room, the kitchen and the fields."

"This rivulet is too far from the pagoda." Phương asked, "You have to spend much money for the pipes, don't you?"

"I split large bamboos to make channels," Vạn Lộc answered. "Bamboo costs nothing. Near the building, I also built a container that supplies enough water for cooking, bathing and washing."

Phương looked at Vạn Lộc with great admiration and fondness.

"What grade have you completed?" Phương asked.

Vạn Lộc laughed, retorting, "Can you guess?"

"Tenth or eleventh grade," Phương tentatively said.

"You're wrong. But I won't say," Vạn Lộc smiled enigmatically. Phương wondered if there was a school nearby, or, maybe he was self-taught.

Phương and Vạn Lộc sat down on a flat stone, and they had glutinous rice steamed with black bean. The novice showed Phuong the chain of hills and mountains that stretched northwest, the farther, the higher.

"This low hill is nearly flat and fertile," Vạn Lộc said. "All the slopes are developed, cultivated, and watered. The pagoda can sustain itself decently."

"You're right," Phương said. "The green fields around here look productive. It is sure that the yield is abundant."

Then Vạn Lộc said, "We should go back to help other novices prepare the altar, because tomorrow is Mid-Autumn celebration, and it'll be a busy day."

Phương passed the night sleepless, obsessed by Vạn Lộc's smiles, and eyes. He wondered why they attracted him too much. They looked like someone's—maybe his mother's. It was strange that Vạn Lộc was sometimes caught looking at him tenderly. Then he slept soundly.

The fifteenth day of the lunar August was a holiday for children and adults. Farmers and their children, in Sunday clothes, gathered on the yard in front of the pagoda before the celebration. They brought sticky rice cakes, moon cakes and colored paper lanterns. The altar was illuminated with candles, and the main hall was filled with incense scent and smoke. The novices were busy arranging flowers and fruits, and lighting candles. Then the prayers began, with the sounds of wooden tocsin and bells. After celebration, the Venerable invited all believers to gather in the dining room to have vegetarian food. The day finished with a procession of paper lantern parade under the bright round moon. Children were very pleased when they went home.

Phương saw Vạn Lộc from time to time, bringing him moon cakes, hot tea, and sticky rice cakes. He wanted to keep Vạn Lộc for a long talk, but Vạn Lộc said that he had to entertain the children, who loved being with him. Phương enjoyed the autumn atmosphere at the pagoda. He looked out through the window to the full moon playing with running clouds, the indistinct moonlight, dancing on the plants in the fields and on the hills. Bamboo tops stood out from the vague black ridge of mountains, swaying with the wind. Haze from the east slowly drifted up and down above the vegetation. He heard crickets chirping everywhere. He used to catch male crickets and let them fight each other. That childhood had passed. Now it was a time when he longed for something, something he could not make out. He felt melancholic and restless.

Early in the morning, Phương woke up as the Morning Prayer resounded into his ears. He came out and sat on a bench in front of the pagoda, looking at the East, the rising sun on the Pacific Ocean. The early hours of the day were like the early years of his life. He was happy to enjoy the first sunrays, the golden clouds, the violet haze in the sky, the waking up of the vegetation, the murmur of the insects, and the monotonous songs of cicadas in the trees. He perceived the bell sound waves shaking the sunrays and the dew curtain. He felt his soul transcending into heavenly happiness. He sensed someone staring at him from behind. He turned his head and saw Vạn Lộc's smiling face. He reached out his hand to hold Vạn Lộc's. But Vạn Lộc lurched aside.

"Hi, what's on your mind? You're delighted, aren't you?" Vạn Lộc asked.

"Hello. Look at that beautiful morning landscape," Phương said. "However, it is missing something, for example, a couple of young . . ."

"Please, don't say that. You're in front of the pagoda," Vạn Lộc flushed.

"I'm sorry . . ."

"Let's have breakfast," Vạn Lộc said. "Then today, I'm going to pick green mung beans on the western hill side. Do you want to go with me?"

"Sure do," Phương replied with a big laugh.

At breakfast, the Venerable met Phương and asked if he was having fun these days. He was very pleased that his nephew loved the countryside, the quiet life in a remote region.

Vạn Lộc gave Phương a bamboo backpack, a bag of glutinous rice, and a bottle of water. They set out to the bean field.

"Make sure you pick the ripe pods, not the young ones," Vạn Lộc said. "Look, those are green, and these are yellow and ripe. Pick them and throw them into the backpack. You won't have your snack until your pack is full, okay?"

"Okay." Both laughed, looking at each other. They competed to pick the most pods, chasing each other between furrows of bean plants. They laughed jovially, showing the biggest pods they could find. However, Vạn Lộc was faster, his backpack was nearly full. Phương followed him. When Vạn Lộc bent over plants to look for pods, Phương stole a handful of pods from Vạn Lộc's backpack and put it into his. On the second time, Vạn Lộc looked up in time and saw Phương's hand full of pods from his backpack.

"Oh, well. You've been caught red-handed," Vạn Lộc said. Phương did not say a word. He just smiled.

"Now. Hands out! Palms up!" Vạn Lộc ordered. He then hit Phương's hands, "One, two, three, four, and .

. . five." Phương tried to catch Van Lộc's hand, but he eluded him.

"I don't feel pain," Phương said. "Your hands are too soft. Here're my hands. Hit them again."

"No. That's enough," Vạn Lộc said, smiling. "Let's go back to the pagoda."

After dinner, Phương sat alone on a bench, watching the sun setting behind the mountain range. The loud song of cicadas, the chirp of crickets, and the darkening of the far away forests covering hills and mountains, kindled Phương's sentiments of melancholy and uneasiness. He felt at a loss as well as needing something. On the top of the range of bamboo bushes, white herons, coming from all directions, gathered and tried to perch, biting, crying and chasing each other, while the black curtain was dropping over the hills. That scene reminded Phương of picking beans this afternoon. It was strange that Vạn Lộc's hands were very smooth, that his voice was clear and soft, and that he showed his shyness at the contact with Phương's hands. Phương had perceived something unusual and weird. The moon had not risen yet. However, feeling sleepy, he drifted asleep.

As soon as Phương awoke, Vạn Lộc came to his mind. He got ready to join him at the breakfast table. There he came to him with a broad charming smile. They ate fried soybean tofu, rice and soybean sauce.

"Here's your bamboo backpack and your snack," the novice said. "We're going to pick tea buds on the southern hill. Today's weather is cool with patchy clouds. We have to keep our eyes open on the weather. There might be a suddenly upcoming shower. This is that kind of autumn day."

"You're always smarter than I am," Phương replied.

From the highest rock, Phương looked down to the river, flowing slowly, embracing the foot of the hill, and then winding far away. Scattered thatched houses bordered the riverbanks. They were built among green rice fields or gardens of fruit trees. Areca trees rose high into the sky like young couples on stilts. Their palm foliages, round like green globes, seemed to be talking to each other as the breeze blew across the countryside.

"Vạn Lộc, how beautiful and picturesque the scene is," Phương said. "Do you feel like I do?"

"Yes, I do," Vạn Lộc slowly agreed, instinctively coming near to Phương, who put an arm around Vạn Lộc's shoulders. Embarrassed, Vạn Lộc got away before Phương's surprised eyes.

"What's the matter with you?" Phương asked.

"Nothing. That's against a religious rule," the novice answered.

"Oh, I'm sorry."

They kept silent, absorbed in picking tea while following their own thinking. Then, they sat down on a stone under a big tree, and had lunch. They looked at each other, smiling and appreciating the taste of sticky cakes that the cook had made. Phương sometimes saw that Vạn Lộc's eyes were far away, lost in his thoughts. Vạn Lộc refused to answer Phương's questions about his family and his past. He said he had forgotten his past and his family. He wanted only to devote himself to the religious life.

"But . . ."

"But what?" Phương asked.

Vạn Lộc stammered, "But there's something . . . boiling in me that I can't sometimes overcome."

"What's that?"

"I won't tell you. Look!" Vạn Lộc said, pointing to the East. "Let's run back to the pagoda. The shower's coming. The proverb says: *Black clouds coming from the East, we have to run as fast as possible. The storm coming from the West, there's only light rain and wind.*"

After dinner, Phương came back to his room. Not long afterwards, there was a knock on the door. He answered it.

"The Venerable offers you some new tea and cookies. He hopes you'll enjoy it," Vạn Lộc said, holding a round china teapot and cups. He put them down on the table, and then poured hot green tea into a cup.

"Please enjoy the tea," the novice said, ready to make for the door.

"No. Don't leave, Vạn Lộc. Sit down and have tea with me," Phương invited.

"No, thanks. I'm busy right now. See you tomorrow morning." Vạn Lộc left the room.

Phương breathed in the fragrant smell of the new tea. Satisfied, he drank it and ate cookies. He then went to sleep. He saw in his dream that Vạn Lộc was a girl, and that both went running up and down the hills, and that he eventually kissed Vạn Lộc. He woke up, happy, but realized that it was ridiculous dream—Vạn Lộc was a boy. He smiled at himself.

The next morning, it was raining hard when Phương was ready for breakfast. The rain slashed through cracks between the windowpanes and under the door. Strong wind blew raindrops across the hallway. It was cloudy, and lightning zigzagged across the black sky. When Phương opened the door, he saw Vạn Lộc bringing breakfast to his room.

"Thank you so much, Vạn Lộc. I think I can go down to the dining room," Phương said.

"The cook doesn't want you to get wet, so he told me to take breakfast to your room," the novice reported.

"The cook's a nice man," Phương said. "Come in and stay for breakfast with me."

"No. Thank you. I had breakfast," Vạn Lộc said. "There are some wet spots in the altar hall. I'm going to dry them. See you later."

After breakfast, Phương had nothing to do. Vạn Lộc did not come. Impatient and restless, Phương walked back and forth in the room. He looked through the glass windowpane, and saw sheets of rain flying by the hills and disappearing down slopes. The wind shook bushes, trees, and bamboo, while bean plants wobbled under the rain. But autumn showers did not last long. At noon, the rain dwindled and died down. The afternoon sun reappeared. Birds and cicadas resumed their songs and the soil started to dry up.

The following was a sunny day. Vạn Lộc, Phương and two other novices went to gather firewood in the forest. They looked for dead fallen trees. They sawed them into two-foot long sections. They chopped and tied them up into bundles that they put into their backpacks. They started going back to the pagoda. Phương and Vạn Lộc could not keep pace with two other novices, they were left far behind. When they came to a shallow muddy stream where they had laid four step-stones to cross it, Phương passed it easily first and waited for Vạn Lộc to cross the brook. Vạn Lộc stepped on the stones. As soon as he put his foot on the fourth step-stone, the rock teetered and Vạn Lộc lost balance and stumbled, going to fall down into the stream. Phương caught his hand and pulled Vạn Lộc hard to him. The pull was so strong and sudden that Vạn Lộc's chest hit Phương's, and Phương embraced Vạn Lộc in his arms. Vạn Lộc reddened and hurried away while Phương was amazed. He murmured, "It's impossible. It's absurd." He tried to forget it, but he couldn't. The sensation was strange. At night, he lay wide-awake, changing positions in the bed. His reason was in conflict with his experience. He remembered the sensation of two hard points pressing on his chest.

The following morning, the novice came smiling at Phương as if nothing had happened. His uncle came to him while he was having breakfast.

"Hi, my dear. How do you like your stay in here?" The Venerable asked.

"Wonderful, Master," Phương answered. "Your pagoda is a peaceful and attractive resort."

"When do you plan to go back home, Phương?"

"The day after tomorrow, Master, because I've been away from home long enough," Phương answered.

"Okay. Enjoy your last days on the hills."

"Thank you, Master," Phương said.

Phương took a quick look at Vạn Lộc, whose countenance changed. The novice got pale and wan. Immediately, a swell of pity mixed with affection for Vạn Lộc came into his heart. He stared into Vạn Lộc's eyes for a while.

Vạn Lộc did not say a word all the way to the field.

"What are we going to do today, Vạn Lộc?" Phương broke the silence.

"Collect eggplants," he answered.

"I'll send you letters regularly when I'm in Saigon," Phương consoled. "I won't forget you, Vạn Lộc."

Vạn Lộc did not reply. Phuong did not know what was on Vạn Lộc's mind. They continued to collect eggplants, lazily.

"You know, Vạn Lộc," Phương said. "My grandma had a big jar of salted eggplants year in and year out. She served salted eggplants to harvesters for their meals during crop seasons."

Vạn Lộc remained silent. Phương had an idea. He looked for a big, one-inch long, dotted worm in an eggplant. He found one, approached Vạn Lộc and threw it to his arm. The novice startled, jumped up, flinging the worm away, and shouted, "You're crazy. I'll beat you." He chased Phương all the way around the field, laughing. When both got tired, they smiled at each other. They came to sit down under a tall guava.

"Have you ever been in those far hills and mountains?" Phương asked.

"No, I haven't," the novice answered. "They are too far away. There could be wild animals."

"Do you want to go with me?" Phương asked.

269

"Where?"

"There, to those hills."

Vạn Lộc looked up at Phương, "What for?"

"For fun."

Vạn Lộc hesitated, then said, "Okay, but wait . . ." He stood up, because he had seen two ripe guavas. He immediately climbed up the tree, and picked them. He ate one and threw the other to Phương.

"Very sweet," Phương said.

Vạn Lộc climbed higher for two more big yellow guavas that were up there. Vạn Lộc was perched, both feet on a branch, his left hand holding an upper branch and his right hand trying to reach the fruit. As soon as he got the guavas, the branch on which he stood broke. He was dangling like a pendulum with his left hand clinging to the branch, which was bending slowly down. He shouted, "Help me, I'm falling!"

"Stay calm! Don't be afraid. I'll catch you," Phương yelled back, his arms straining out and his legs wide apart. Phương looked up at Vạn Lộc falling down onto him. He caught Vạn Lộc in his robust arms. Vạn Lộc's body was so heavy that it pulled Phương down forcing him to sit on the ground. The impact on Phương's arms was so strong that Vạn Lộc fainted, and the upper buttons of Vạn Lộc's robe detached. The robe flaps broadly opened and one white female breast stuck out. Phương was surprised, his eyes and mouth were wide open. However, to be sure, he lifted the other flap, and he saw the other breast. Suddenly, he felt extremely happy. He muttered slowly and quietly, "Vạn Lộc is a girl. That's what I have dreamed of." He bent his head down wanting to tenderly kiss, as Vạn Lộc recovered her consciousness. She was at a loss what to say or what to do. Her eyes welled in tears.

"Are you all right?" Phương asked. "Don't move! Are you all right? Tell me where you feel pain."

"My legs and heels hurt," she said. Phương smiled at her while he soothingly massaged her legs, and then her heels. Vạn Lộc hid her emotions, turning away her eyes.

"What's your real name?" Phương asked, after a long moment.

"Thu," she said, and implored. "Please keep this secret for me. If not, I must leave the pagoda. I don't know where to go. I do not have any relative in this city. Nobody except you knows this secret, not even the Master."

"Okay! I promise," Phương said.

"I'll tell you my past and my secrets one day," Thu said.

Phương helped Thu stand up and they walked back to the pagoda.

Phương passed that night wakeful, wrapped up in thoughts of Thu.

Phương did not meet Thu the next day. She was in bed the whole day. The cook brought her meals. Phương was anxious and worried. He wanted to see her in her room, but her door was locked. He wondered if she got better, and what he could do to help her and to be near her. He was restless the whole day.

On the eve of his departure, Phương was agitated, walking back and forth in his room. He looked out through the window—outside was black. Crickets chirped everywhere. Cicadas sang noisily and monotonously in the trees. He wandered through the door to the back yard. Everyone slept soundly. The entire pagoda was black. He took a good look at the pagoda panorama at night, the surrounding hills and the far mountains. He wanted to fix these images in his memory. Then he sat down on a bamboo bench.

Suddenly, a soft hand lay down on his shoulder. He held it, knowing whose hand it was.

"I miss you, and I love you, Thu," Phương said.

"You can't marry me because your mother won't let you," Thu said. "As an orphan, I know my condition, my destiny."

"Don't worry," Phương replied. "My mother loves me very much. I can persuade her about our marriage."

After a moment of silence, Thu continued, "I was torn between my devotion to the religious life, and my love for you—that I can't overcome. Images of you obsess my mind, day and night. I'm crazy about you."

"I promise to marry you, Thu. Take my word," Phương said.

A hare sprang out of a bush and ran into its hole. Thu shuddered and Phương embraced her, kissing her cheeks, then on the mouth. She was shivering with emotion rather than a chill. Small yellow glistening fireflies flew around them. It seemed that they cheered the young lovers. Two white rabbits raced out of their hole, trying to mate or looking for food. It was midnight when the autumn moon rose from the East and shone fitfully between ragged clouds. Thu, her hands clasped in his, was too moved, too emotional to talk for a time.

"Do you really love me, Phương?" Thu asked. "I can't bear a day without you."

"I love you, and I will marry you, Thu," Phương an-
swered.

When Phương and Thu went back to their rooms,
the moon was very round, and shone in the dark-blue sky.
Phương watched Thu walking in the moonlight, until
she disappeared into her room.

After breakfast, Phương went to the Master's room
and said good-bye to his uncle. The Master told him to
say "hello" to his sister for him and to come back next
summer for another vacation. He said goodbye to other
novices and the cook. Vạn Lộc had excused himself for
illness. Phương went down the trail with broken-heart-
ed emotions. On the train, he slept the entire journey to
Saigon. His mother was happy to hear of her brother's
health and the peaceful hills he lived on. Phương felt
happy to live in the ambience of his mother's happiness
as well. But the following week, images of Thu flooded
his mind. He was eager to see her again.

Three weeks later, he came back to the familiar and
beloved hills, with his mother's letter to the Venerable.
His uncle was glad to read his sister's letter, and agreed to
let Vạn Lộc go to Saigon to teach his sister Buddhist doc-
trine. Vạn Lộc said good-bye to the Master, other nov-
ices, and the cook. They both went down to the horse-
cart stop at the end of the trail. Phương gave Thu civilian
clothes and a female wig that she put on, behind some
bushes.

"Thu, you know I love you and want to marry you,"
Phương said. "Mom accepted our marriage."

"Thank you, Phương," replied Thu. "My father was
shot dead, following a failed coup d'état against the

French domination. My mom was afraid and fled Hànội, taking me to a village near the pagoda. But when I was ten, mom could not survive her illness. Before she passed away, she had disguised me as a boy and took me to the pagoda. She told the Venerable that she would not live any longer because of the sickness, and she begged the Master to take me as a Buddhist novice after her death. I had lived there at the pagoda ever since. I wanted my complete devotion to a religious life, until I met you."

She said, "The more I know of you, Phương, the more I love you. I cannot concentrate on my morning and evening prayers. I have found that love is stronger than religious devotion. I want to be held, to be loved, and to be protected. I am an orphan, so I need love. The day I fell from the guava tree and you held me in your arms, your male warmth went into my veins, my heart, and my soul. Devotion to the religious life is wonderful, but love is better."

"I hold you now . . . and forever, Thu," Phưng said, as they embraced.

A Bus Ride

"Honey! Don't wait for me next month," Đính said to Phan, her husband.

"When'll you come?" Phan asked.

"The first day of December, my dear. I think you have enough food for two months."

"Okay. Take care. Please tell our children, 'I love them and I miss them' for me, sweet-heart."

"Yes, I will. Don't forget to take vitamins every day."

"No, I won't. Bye, Đính," Phan said, tenderly pressing her hands and passionately looking into her eyes, as if he wanted his love to enter her soul.

She watched Phan leaving her, walking slowly, carrying heavily, a bamboo pole on his shoulder, the bag of rice she had brought hung on one end of the pole, the bag of food on the other end. Her gaze followed his skeleton-like body, his hollow-cheeked dark-tanned face, his sunken, haggard eyes. She had sold all his Sunday best—dark mohair suits, plain white polyester shirts, black Italian leather shoes, and chic French-styled ties. She had brought instead, the *Relief for Refugees* pants and shirts he was now wearing. She felt the burden of the bags he was carrying pounding on her shrinking heart. A bitter lump swelled and thickened in her throat while Phan's profile was dwindling among green cassava fields. The picture of a victorious officer of the South Vietnam Army, her husband, was now nothing but a wretchedly deplorable prisoner. There was no more dignity of human beings. The fall of South Vietnam shattered the free Vietnamese's families, husbands imprisoned in the jungle, and dying from hunger, labor, and torture; children thrown into the streets, waiting for leftovers at the front of the cheap restaurants; wives selling their belongings. Lots of wives and children were coerced to move to the new economic zones, where each family was given a hooch (improvised shelter) and a small piece of land to plant cassava. That was the fate of the defeated freedom fighters.

Remembering her return trip, Đính ran out of the waiting-house and hurried onto the road to catch the bus. She heard the driver's helper shouting, "Hold on!

Hold on! Uncle Tám, one more woman's coming!" The bus, which had just started rolling a few yards, came to a stop.

Đính arrived at the back of the van, panting. The helper looked into the bus.

"Any room in this row?" He asked.

As one, all the women protested, "Ten persons in this row."

The helper searched the middle row. A large woman protested, "I'm sitting only on half of my behind."

He looked into the left row. At that moment, the driver yelled to the helper, "Put her up here. She can sit with the boy." Đính got on the bus and sat beside the door. The boy's mother was between him and Đính. The bus took off. Although the passengers were not entirely comfortable in their seats, they felt relieved having left the undesirable hostile area, as they had been reluctant to come, because it was confining their beloved.

These women were the wives of former South Vietnamese government officials or army officers. They had come the previous day, and passed the night in the thatched waiting-house of Bà Tô political prison. Bà Tô was a small village about 30 miles north of Vũng Tàu, Vietnam. The jail had ten wooden houses covered with fan-palm leaves, they were built after the April 30, 1975 surrender to the Việt Cộng. The jail, far from the populated area, was at the edge of a forest and near a stream. The political prisoners were allowed to meet their wives and children, and to receive food and rice only on the first day of the month.

"Why are you so late, Đính?" a middle-aged woman asked in a Huế accent. "You've almost missed the bus."

"My husband has been sick, Hai," Đính answered. "He's as pale as a young banana leaf. I had a hard time seeing him off."

"So is my husband," the woman confided. "He was as strong as a water buffalo. Now, he's so thin and so bony. What a pity!"

"Prisoners are fed with nothing but cassava (manioc) powder all the year round," Đính explained.

"You know," the woman with two dimples on her cheeks said, "cassava that is not properly processed is hazardous to human health."

"Did you bring rice and meat to your husband?" A large woman in a black blouse asked.

"Yes, and I brought him vitamins and medicine, too," Đính answered.

All these women, Đính thought, had the same anxiety, the same survival concerns: their husbands' health, how to earn money, and how to ensure their children's food and education. Her savings had drained to zero following the change of currency, 500 dongs (Vietnamese currency) for one new dong, the maximum of exchangeable money being limited to two hundred thousand old dongs, so the rest of their fortune had become waste paper. Her house, like the other women's, became almost empty of furniture and house wares, sold to eke out a living. There were no jobs, because factories were closed or confiscated.

Their tiredness, and the monotonous sound of the bus engine made the women fall asleep easily. Each woman's head bent against the next woman's shoulder or against the bus body. Some started to snore loudly. But Đính could not close her eyes, her mind reeling off successive pictures from the wonderful wedding days to the Black Day of April 30, 1975. The sudden shock of losing her happiness, her family comfort and welfare, and her children's future was hurting her soul, leaving a wound that deepened and deepened.

It was the first day of October, a sunny day. The sun was shining on dark-green rubber trees on the left-hand side of the road. Đính did not see any rubber-workers collecting latex. Some rubber trees had empty coconut hardshells, but most of the trees had lost them. The furrows carved around the trunks, along which the latex used to run down to the bowls, had dried off, leaving sad, cold, and brown scars. Fields of cassava were on the right-hand side. There were no rice paddies in this area. Some naked children, who showed their big round bellies, stood in front of their empty thatched huts, scattered in the so-called new economic zone.

The rainy season was ending. Looking in the rear mirror, Đính saw red dust fly high, and spread in all directions, making a big red moving cloud, blocking her view. The bus ran smoothly at the speed of only twenty miles per hour. Suddenly, Đính heard steel clanging below her seat, and she saw a wheel run off, alongside the bus and then into a ditch. Not perceiving the peril, she was surprised at what was going on before her eyes. By instinct, she uttered, "Hey! Driver! A wheel is rolling off into the ditch." On quick second thoughts, she said, "Be careful. Slow down gradually or the bus will overturn." The driver, an experienced one, calmly slowed down. As soon as the bus came to a stop, it leaned over to the right front side, and plowed a three-foot long rut. The bus was shaking strongly, as if it were bouncing on a stony pot-holed surface. Passengers, awakened from their sleep, panicked, and shouted "What's happening, Driver?"

"What's the matter with you, Driver?"

"Oh, My goodness! Accident?" A large woman cried.

Đính opened the bus door, got off, and felt at ease. The driver said, "Please, all of you, ladies, get off the van. We're going to fix it."

The women crowded at the front of the bus. They were lucky and happy that they had just escaped an accident. A helper brought back the wheel from the ditch and another helper took down a spare wheel from the bus roof. He also brought out a toolbox and a hydraulic jack. The driver asked the passengers to give a push to the bus to balance it. Observing the five bolts on the wheel-disk, Đính knew why the wheel had come off: the bolt threads were worn down. Because of tire shortages, one of the four tires that had a two-inch long cut, was patched from the inside with four hexagonal nuts on both sides. That was why the bus had traveled slowly. The van was a French-made Renault, transformed into a passenger bus. The two back doors had been taken off and replaced by an eight-millimeter steel chain. In the bus, two one-foot wide, pinewood benches were fixed to the sides of the body. The middle bench, in wood too, was removable, to allow transportation of bulky produce. Đính looked at a cylindrical black steel tank about four feet high and one and half feet in diameter, welded vertically onto the right side of the rear of the bus. There was a round opening at the bottom of the tank, where red-hot charcoal was burning. Because gasoline was in desperately short supply, people had to use charcoal to power vehicles. After one hour or so of repair work, the passengers got on the bus, expecting they would be home soon. Then the bus drove past brick houses on the asphalt streets of Bà Rịa City. The bus stopped at the bus station near Bà Rịa fish market. The women went shopping. Seafood was fresh and cheap. Đính saw rows of rusty, bullet-holed sheet-metal covered stalls beside weather-beaten brick kiosks on a large market ground. She looked at the seafood stands. In a flat basket, three hand-palm-sized crabs were tied with reed around their claws and legs, their mouth puffing water bubbles. A smiling, middle-age woman advertised her ear-shaped abalones, three of them about four inches in length, with others smaller. A young woman, about 30, invited Đính to buy her round fat tuna. Showing a six-pound tuna in a hand scale, she said the fish was very fresh by indicating its red gills. A teenage boy had green and white mussels displayed on his wooden stand. Đính bought three abalones and two live crabs. She walked to the fruit section, which did not have shelter because it was the seasonal produce location. An old man wearing a blue worn-out shirt and black pants, had some big jackfruit lying on the ground and a basket of durians. Yellowish tangerines and grapefruit with green leaves at the stems were fresh, and attractively delicious. A little girl had a small basket of reddish yellow pomegranates. Đính bought one large jackfruit. She wanted to purchase more, but she could not afford it.

Coming back to the bus, she saw the helpers were busy covering dozens of five-gallon cans of fish sauce with a large tarp on the bus roof. Next to the tin cans, stacks of firewood bundles were tightened with coco ropes to the rail welded on the bus roof. There was a lot of firewood under the seat benches as well. The passengers had to step on them to sit down. They felt very uncomfortable, but they restrained their anger, as they had been doing it for many years under the Communist regime. They had no choice.

The women were pleased with what they had bought because of the cheap price and the freshness. Đính heard them talk to each other.

"Kim, you've got a fat tuna. How much is it?" A pretty woman asked her friend.

"Look, Tu. It's fresh and very cheap. It cost only two dongs and it weighs almost six pounds," Kim replied. "I have to pay double that in Saigon."

"What else did you buy?" Tư asked.

"I bought two lobsters, five crabs, and five pounds of green mussels. How about you?"

"One jackfruit, two durians, and a five-pound tuna," answered Tư, about 40, clad in a light purple blouse and faded grey slacks.

"You have well chosen that jackfruit. Look at its spines. They are very sparse: that means the pulp is soft, thick, and sweet," Kim said.

Đính was content when the bus pulled out of the bus station and into Vũng Tàu Highway. The cool breeze coming from the sea was blowing into the bus, caressing her face. The sunlight was oblique in the West. Rice paddies were very green on both sides of the highway. It seemed to her that farmers in the rice fields were tired and indifferent. When Đính's bus passed, they stood up, smiling at the passengers in the bus while others were gathering their stuff, ready to go home. It was four p.m. on Đính's watch. Young couples in colored tops and pants, riding their Honda motorcycles, parties of two or three mopeds, overtook Đính's bus. Their wives or girl friends on the back of the bikes were waving toward her, showing their sunburned smiling faces. Their happiness was contagious. Đính shared it, sensing the outside world was still having some aspects worthy of living. In an instant she forgot her misery, thinking of her children's brilliant future.

Đính's bus was about two miles from Long Thành City, famous for its orchards of durian, grapefruit, and jackfruit. A long blue bus crowded with passengers and loaded with merchandise on the roof, coming toward them, was flashing its headlights. A helper standing at the back of the on-coming bus made some signs to the helpers of her bus. Đính did not understand their meaning.

Suddenly, Đính heard a helper hit the bus body twice and shout, "Uncle Tám, FSA ahead!"

"I've got it," the driver replied. Then he slowed down the bus and made a U-turn. All the passengers protested loudly.

"What the hell's going on, Driver?" An aggressive woman shouted.

"My God, why did you make a U-turn?" An old lady asked, harshly.

"It's getting late. I have to go home early. My kids have been left at home for two days. I don't know what happened to them."

The driver and the helpers kept their mouths shut.

"Why did you make a U-turn, Uncle Tám?" Đính softly asked the driver. "What does FSA stand for?"

"The FSA stands for Forest Service Agents. They are stationed somewhere near Long Thành City. You know, the bus spare parts are rare and expensive these days. I buy them on the black market. The new government does not import them. So I deliver firewood or charcoal to have some extra money. If I get caught, the firewood or the charcoal will be confiscated, and I have to pay its owner for it."

"When'll the agents go home?" Đính asked.

"I'll wait until about six p.m.," Uncle Tám said. "It's about time they were off duty. Besides, I pay many taxes, and I have to bribe the Highway Patrol Policemen by either money or "555" cigarette packs."

"It's six-oh-five now. You can take off, Uncle Tám," Đính said.

When the bus arrived at Long Thành, firewood was taken down. The women felt satisfied, but it did not last long. Boy and girl peddlers crowded around the bus, selling drinks and food. They were barefooted, wearing shabby black clothes and yelling all the time.

"Hot tea! Ten-cents a glass!" shouted a skinny, suntanned-faced girl, about 12.

Đính bought a glass of hot tea and drank it. To the passengers' surprise, bags of charcoal were loaded onto the top of the bus. Coal dust flew over Đính's and passengers' heads, but everyone was too tired to complain. They used hands or towels to fan coal dust away, grumbling. Đính knew that the passengers' protest had no impact on the driver and his helpers, who were used to it.

When the charcoal was well piled up on the roof, and the electric lights around the Long Thành City were on, the driver drove the van onto the road. Passengers sighed with relief. Đính looked through the bus windows. It was dark on both sides of the road because of the tree foliage. Afar, appeared, then disappeared dots of light, going up and down like dancing phosphorescent fires.

"Looks like white ghosts," Đính said to the woman beside her, pointing to the light dots.

"Maybe they are dead soldiers' souls, trying to find a way home. Some soldiers were shot dead and their bodies were buried in a hurry. Their relatives do not know where their tombs are," the woman answered. Đính felt scared as well as painful because a surge of pain from her heart to her eyes made her tears come out and run down her cheeks.

"Those women back there and we are lucky, because your husband, mine, and theirs are still alive," she continued. "The majority of women of our generations are widows. That God-damned war, and we were defeated."

Đính looked back to other women's faces. She saw in the dim light their eyes traveling far away. It seemed that they had the same feeling as Đính did.

"Some old women had buried their husbands before the 1954 Geneva Treaty," Đính said. "They then buried their sons and daughters during the 1973 Paris

Agreement, and finally they fled Vietnam to the United States, empty-handed, with their nephews and nieces after 1975. They lost everything: husbands, children, furnished houses, lands, and savings in the banks. Those cruel Communist thieves!"

Suddenly, the bus dropped into a deep dip. All the women came back to reality. It was near Long Bình, the former USAID logistics compound.

"Stop the bus!" A woman shrieked, "Fish sauce!"

"Fish sauce's dripping!" Another yelled.

The helpers looked toward the direction of the shouts. They asked, "What's the matter, ladies?"

The women on one side of the bus said at the same time, "Fish sauce's dripping."

Then they cursed the driver. They all stood up and shouted, "Driver, stop the bus!"

The bus stopped. They got off and yelled to the driver, pointing to their fish-sauce-stained blouses and to the line of sauce running down the bus.

"Look, fish sauce on my blouse."

"There, it's dripping."

"How can I wash it off my blouse?"

The driver did not reply. He knew that silence would buy forgiveness. He said to one helper, "Get up to the roof and put the broken can into this plastic bag." He then told the other helper, "Take a can and get water from that pond." The helper also cleaned fish sauce from the bus. The women washed their blouses and kept on cursing the driver, the helpers, and the bus, saying, "What a bad day! What a damned bus!"

At last, the driver begged them to get on the bus. The bus rolled onto Sàigòn-Biên-Hòa Highway and ran smoothly, without incident, to the bus station.

Đính got on a tricycle at the Saigon Eastern bus station.

"Where to, ma'am?" The cyclo man asked.

"Trần Hưng Đạo Boulevard, please."

"O my God! Do you smell fish sauce?" He asked.

"No, I don't," she lied.

Edna Woolley

Edna is both versatile and eclectic. In our workshops, she has written two novellas, as well as her memoirs, examples of which follow. All of the workshop writers produce scenes that are unforgettable, and it seems to me that none is more so than Edna's account of going to a picture show (namely, "The Jazz Singer") with her mother.

—W.R.W.

One Remarkable Woman

This is a story about my remarkable mother. I'm sure you would agree that any woman who bore nineteen children, no multiples, deserves this title from that fact alone, but my story gives additional strength to this claim.

Born December 8, 1886, Vada Ellen Hurlbut, married my father, Henry William Maisenbach, August 16, 1905 and eventually gave him eight boys and eleven girls. Though small of stature at five-feet-three-inches tall, Mom's health never failed to meet the needs of her small figure, and the smile she gave when speaking to you, revealed a constant inner peace. She loved hold-

287

ing and nursing each and every baby and spent endless hours bonding with them. I remember observing the sparkle in her eyes as she gazed lovingly into their eyes. It was then that I knew she adored all of her babies.

We lived in the small town of Muscatine in the Southeastern part of Iowa, a town located on the Mississippi River, also known as "Pearl City." It was given that name because the pearl-button industry that flourished there. My father's employment for most of his married life was in a small shop on the outskirts of town, where he worked as a skilled button cutter in addition to making fashion accessories. He was a loving father who was dedicated to providing for our health and happiness, never missing a day of work, so I have good memories of him also, but this story is dedicated to Mom.

Yes, we were deprived in many ways because of the size of our family, but because of the Great Depression, other families suffered deprivations along with us. So did various businesses affected by the loss of activity during the darkness of the depression, not to mention the schools we attended. Though we were deprived, we were no more aware of deprivation than others living in our town.

In our home, there were few opportunities for family entertainment aside from the games we played, and later, music and shows from radio. That is the reason that this particular time stands out in my memory, for this is the story of the unusual strength and determination of our mother and the unusual gift of the memory she inadvertently gave to me, the oldest of the last six of her children. This experience is stamped in my memory now, especially, as it relates not only to an exceptional experience many others in our town failed to enjoy, but also to those in the world who missed the opportunity.

Mom was expecting her eighteenth baby in November. No one knew her secret, of course, because she always wore dresses that hung loosely from her shoulders, a scheme she used to fool our neighbors so she could spring the arrival of a new baby on them. Her ruse always worked, except for her eighteenth baby, born breech—butt first, that is, and she had to go to our nearby community hospital. The rest were born at home.

I was her fourteenth child, born July 28, 1922, named Edna Ruth, and at five years of age, was the oldest of a group of four treated to a special outing. Jo Ann Margaret was four; Phyllis Mae was three; and Iva Jean, the baby, was not quite a year old. It was the year 1927, and Mom had gathered us together on this special day, and said to me, "Edna, please help me get the others ready. We're going to a movie." I didn't know what a movie was, but I became extremely excited because we were going "out," and the thought of that alone was exciting. I realize now that Mom had never been to a movie before, but I recall overhearing her tell a neighbor that this was the very first movie produced with sound "the greatest historical achievement in the entertainment world," and she wasn't going to miss it.

It was over a mile to the Palace Theatre, so she placed the baby in her "ancient wicker-buggy;" I say ancient because, as I remember, the body of the buggy was made of a hand-woven wooden-basket-weave, and the huge, oversized wheels were made of iron, covered in hard rubber, which was worn so thin that the exposed metal rims clanged loudly on the pavement as they turned (I'm sure now, that that buggy was used for all nineteen of her babies). We followed closely beside our mother, tripping eagerly along, heading for we knew not what. I don't know how she managed this adventure because she was again over seven months pregnant, her loose dress managing to hide her pregnancy from the eyes of "nosey neighbors."

At the theater, she pushed the buggy forward with the determination of one who believed firmly "nothing ventured, nothing gained." She shoved it to the open theatre door, turned it around and backed it up the two steps and through the door, and then parked it against the wall inside the entry. She swept Iva Jean up in her arms, marched to the ticket window and handed the ticket-lady fifteen cents to purchase her ticket. The ticket-lady's eyes widened as she gasped in surprise, and raised her arms in the air, her ten fingers spread apart in alarm as she looked at the sight of the baby in Mom's arms and what probably looked like a small brigade of little ones trailing behind her. We kids didn't need tickets. Mom hurried us to the "little girls" room, then made sure we all "pee-peed."

As we left the rest room, the pungent smell of freshly popped corn permeated the atmosphere of the hallway, and the girl attending the popcorn-popper stared at us intently.

We three children stopped abruptly, staring up in astonishment at the sound of the popper exploding the popcorn, our eyes bulging in amazement and our noses wrinkling at the delicious smell, and in anticipation looked up at Mom with pleading eyes. Mom, balancing the baby in one arm, quickly searched in her handbag and found a nickel. She bought one huge bag of lusciously buttered popcorn, and handed the bag to me. Then she proceeded into the theater, leading us down the aisle to about the fifth row from the front.

"I'll take the aisle seat in case the baby gets fussy," she whispered to me as she sat down, placing Iva Jean, on her lap (though she didn't have much of a lap because her stomach was so swelled from her seven-months' pregnancy) and we all piled in on the other side of her. I sat in the middle of the two younger ones, tightly gripping the bag of popcorn as if my life depended on it, each of us gulping down the popcorn and quickly digging for more. This was our first experience with popcorn, and it was delicious. The lights were on when we sat down, but after a few minutes, they were extinguished, and the theatre was engulfed in stark blackness! We all became startled and frightened, and began protesting at the sudden change, but Mom quieted us with a finger to her lips and in a loud whisper, instructing us: "Shush! . . . It's okay . . . the movie's starting."

Suddenly, the blare of deafening music filled the theatre, then the curtains were drawn apart, and the words: "Warner Brothers—Supreme Triumph—Al Jolson in THE JAZZ SINGER" filled the screen. I will never forget the high pitch of Mom's voice as, in her excitement, she let out a loud gasp, OH! . . . MY! . . . at the overpowering sound of the background music during the introduction of the movie. This was the very first moving picture produced with sound. I was too young to realize the significance—but I do remember—Al Jolson, perched on one knee, his arms outstretched to his little boy, his rich, resonant voice singing out, "Climb upon my knee . . . Sonny Boy."

Mom, her own baby on her lap, began to sob. . . ."OH, MY! . . . this is so, beautiful." Iva Jean, asleep, began to scream at the sounds of Mom's loud exclamations and the loud reverberations of sounds throbbing in the theatre. Mom quickly quenched her sobs, wiped her flood of tears on her sleeve, and began rocking her, cuddling her closely, humming softly in her ear, until she again fell asleep. I still remember wondering why my mother was crying. I thought the music and Al Jolson's singing was beautiful, not realizing the significance of the fact that this was not only the introduction of the first "talkie," but the first movie musical with the additionally beauty of Al Jolson's voice set to music. I later learned, that Georgie Jessel, who played the role on Broadway, was signed to reprise it on film, but he had a major disagreement with Warner Brothers, and Al Jolson won the film role.

This was the only movie I ever recall my mother attending, but she was determined not to miss this event, and had it not been for her, I would have missed the experience. This is one of the best, if not my favorite, memory of my mother. On November 27, 1927, about two months after this experience, Mom gave birth to

William Donald, our youngest brother, the breech baby. On January 20, 1929 Myrna Eileen, her nineteenth and final child, was born at home. Even more startling is the fact that her first baby was born December 13, 1905, and the last one was born on January 20, 1929, meaning she had nineteen children in a space of twenty-three years—no multiples—all separate births.

My mother's father, Allen Jonathon Hulbut, born November 2, 1853, and blind shortly after birth, died March 1, 1928, at the age of seventy-five years. Grandma, Mary Ellen Hurlbut, born October 4, 1866, was his dedicated wife and mother of his five children. Together, they also raised and nurtured two great-grand-children. Ten years after his death, in 1938, our maternal grandmother came to live with us, and lived another fifteen years, bedridden and requiring full-time care. After giving birth to nineteen children, and seeing her last child marry in 1950, Mom cared for her mother until she died November 22, 1953, at the age of eighty seven from a stroke. Perhaps my grandparents were the role models of strength and determination, which influenced my mother's own strength and determination.

In 1960, my parents moved to Orange, California, to live with Jo Ann (number 15), who never married. My father lived to be eighty. My mother lived to be eighty-eight, eventually requiring colostomy surgery from which she never recovered. For years, she had been suffering from an overactive bowel, which caused diarrhea, for which her doctor put her on a no-rough-age diet. As a result, her bowel became impacted and ruptured, requiring a colostomy. She survived, but remained in a coma, from which she never recovered, soon dying of a stroke. If the doctor hadn't put her on the diet, there's no telling how long she might have lived. Both my parents lived in California until their deaths, and both of their bodies were shipped back to Muscatine, Iowa, and buried in the family plot.

I am convinced that, considering all the circumstances, my mother was indeed: "One Remarkable Woman."

Molly's Folly

It was a hot summer day, one of those days in the Midwest where most grade-school children begin to experience a sadness that only they can understand. Summer vacation was almost over, and like most children on the block, we began to think of using each day left to the fullest. Little did I know that it would be a special day in my life for I would soon learn the true meaning of the word "thankfulness." I was only twelve at the time of this adventure, but if it hadn't been for the gift of God's love in my life, I could have suffered the grief of contributing to the death of my youngest brother, Billy.

Next door to me lived a boy named Hubert Snell. He was a thirteen-year-old boy known for his ability to spark up the lives of every child in the neighborhood when fun ran low. Hubert was born with "the luck of the Irish" as his mother always insisted, despite the fact that he could sometimes create problems no Irish kid would ever dare to give his mother. Regardless of his reputation in the past, without Hubert to rely on, our lives would have been extremely dull at times.

As I said, our summer vacation from school was almost over, and we were "all ears," when Hubert suggested an exciting adventure to give us "something to remember for the rest of our lives." However, Hubert's promises didn't always give him the same ring of truth as you will see as you read my story.

What kid doesn't love horses? Hubert came up with a plan to catch the interest of the most disinterested kid on the block, but we lived next door to him, so we were always the first ones he approached with his "plans."

Hubert claimed he knew where we could go horseback riding, and it wouldn't cost us a cent, because it was a secret place only he knew about. He promised we would have lots of fun hiking to the country to get there. He said he had discovered a beautiful horse out there, and no other kid in the neighborhood knew about her but him.

My little brother, Billy, who was only seven, Phyllis, who was nine, and me, twelve at the time, immediately became interested. We had never been allowed to go that far away from home before, but both of our parents were working, and just the thought of hiking to the country was exciting. We were eager for the adventure, not giving it a thought that there might be dire consequences to pay if anything disastrous happened as a consequence.

The sun was blistering hot, and as was usually the case, the sidewalks absorbed the heat to the fullest.

Nevertheless, we began the trek to the country hot on the heels of Hubert.

During the summer we always went without shoes, so our feet were calloused, but on this day, we had to hop back and forth from the grass to the sidewalk to keep from blistering our feet. Finally, we had covered almost two miles, and the sidewalk abruptly ended. We followed Hubert across a hard, mud-packed path, resulting probably from recent rains in the area, and packed down from Hubert's own feet in the past. Finally, we entered a thicket of dried grass and thistles. As we trudged through the thistles, the down of the ripe flower-heads wafted up around us, carried upward from the ground by the action of our feet and a soft, gentle wind helping them to rise above our heads. Now, suddenly, we realized we were in the country. Trees bordered the path, and ahead of us, we could see the abrupt curve of a hillside over which Hubert led us, and which overlooked a beautiful meadow below. Beyond, we could barely see the faint outlines of a corral and an adjoining red barn. Suddenly, we knew this was the beginning of our great adventure.

Looking down the hill, we could see the tall, golden grass of the meadow, curving and bending from the occasional sweep of the wind. All we had to do now was to descend this steep hill, run across the meadow, and we would reach the corral. Hand in hand, we descended the hill and ran screaming across the meadow towards the corral. As we approached the corral, we could see the most beautiful chestnut-colored mare we had ever seen, and we could hear her whinny as she thrust her head up and down, greeting Hubert. It was clear she knew him. Reaching the corral, we noticed she wore a long, flowing mane, the color of freshly-pulled taffy, and she immediately pranced over to greet us, turning her head and rubbing her neck against the rail as though asking to be stroked. Hubert reached over the rail and patted her on the cheek.

"Hi there, Molly," he said. She shook her head up and down and whinnied in greeting. We could see she was well-fed and cared for, and her wide back glistened in the sunlight as though she had recently been groomed. Not only was her back broad, but her chest was full and well-developed. Her eyes were large, the pupils were a deep, reddish-brown, matching her coat, and she had long eyelashes that half-covered her eyes. We knew it was a special privilege to have a ride on a horse such as this, and each of us waited excitedly as Hubert proceeded to get the bridle, which he had hidden in the stump of a nearby tree. He had very carefully covered it with leaves and dirt so only he would know where it was each time he returned. He told us we would have to ride bareback though, as there was no saddle.

He carried the bridle in one hand and walked over to the corral rail. "Lookie here, Molly," he said, as he reached in his pocket and pulled out a big, red apple, holding it in his outstretched palm beneath the horse's nose. She opened her mouth, and he pushed the apple between her teeth. He quickly climbed over the rail as she chomped on the apple and slipped the bridle over her head, adjusting the metal bit in her mouth before she finished the apple. We could see he knew exactly what he was doing, then he quickly positioned the leather straps of the bridle over her head, and grasping the reins, he pulled them down in front of her head and led her to the gate. He unlatched the gate, and Molly pranced outward toward us. It was clear she needed to be exercised and was looking forward to a good run.

Billy could hardly stand still. He was rather small for his age, and was really not a child of robust health. He was the eighteenth child in our family of nineteen children, small of stature but full of self-confidence and exuberance, and at a time like this, nothing mattered. He began jumping up and down. "I wan'ta be first . . . I wan'ta be first," he cried, excitedly.

Hubert grabbed him and hoisted him up on Molly's back, and before Hubert had a chance to give Billy the reins, Molly took off like a flash. The reins flew aimlessly in the air, and Billy grabbed onto that beautiful, long mane. He instinctively clutched his short legs tightly around the horse's broad back as she dashed off, heading in the direction of the hill we had just descended. Billy began screaming in terror, wildly hanging on desperately to her mane. Molly had just ascended the hill a short distance, but then turned abruptly, heading back down the steep hill. We were all screaming, "Hang on, Billy. Hang on!" Still clinging to her mane, his small body slipped off her back and flew around to the front of her neck, hanging down between her two front legs. He finally lost his grip on the mane, but luckily, when he lost his grip he slipped down between her two front legs and fell quickly to the ground.

Molly continued down the hill without even touching our little brother's body. We were all so thankful he wasn't hurt that we ran immediately up the hill to him. He was crying out in fright, but after quieting him, the scare was enough warning, and we were ready to leave for home—right now!

Molly dashed back to the corral, but Hubert, grabbing the reins, quickly hoisted himself up on Molly's back. "I didn't come all this way without getting my ride," he yelled, as Molly again headed for the hill. This time, halfway up the hill, she again turned abruptly and headed back down. It all happened so quickly that Hubert wasn't prepared and slipped off her back, hitting the ground with a terrible thud. Unfortunately, he wasn't as lucky as Billy. He got up, holding his arm and screaming in extreme pain. He then immediately wanted to go home. Molly had returned to the corral, and Hubert realized he had to first remove the bridle and put it back in the tree stump. He could only use one arm to open the gate, put Molly back inside, and remove the bridle. It took a lot of effort, but he finally hid it back in the stump again and covered it up, groaning in pain all the while.

Just as we started to leave, we saw a man coming in our direction. He waved his arm to get our attention, and as he came up to us, he said, "Is your father home?" Our family was well-known in town, I was scared stiff, thinking he was going to tell our father on us. Thinking quickly, I said, "No, he had to go out of town today."

"Okay," said the man, "I'll come see him later."

Now, we really had to hurry home, I thought, to get there before our folks got home from work. "Let's go, kids," I said, "we've got to get home before that man gets there to tell on us."

All the way home, Hubert moaned and groaned, complaining about his arm, and after awhile, he really started to cry out in pain, the tears streaming down his face. He told us later that his mother really lit into him because she had to take him to a doctor. It turned out his arm was broken, and consequently he couldn't deliver his newspapers—she had to deliver them for him! Just the luck of the Irish, I guess!

As it turned out, the man that we had talked to at the corral wasn't the owner of the farm who was going to tell our father on us. He was some man who wanted to talk to the farmer who owned the farm, whom he thought was our father. When he didn't show up to talk with our father, is when it finally dawned on me. As a child, you think like a child, I guess!

I was so thankful that Billy wasn't killed by Molly trampling on him, that I resolved never to get involved in Hubert Snell's plans again. Many years had passed when one day I asked my mother whatever happened to Hubert, she said that when he got older he was constantly in trouble with the law, and eventually served some time in prison. Incidentally, we never told our parents about our folly with Molly.

What Fun It Was

Looking back to my early childhood days, when I was nine, I remember a snowfall of an especially wonderful Iowa winter. It was early morning and, from my perfect vantage point behind the living room windows, I could not tell where the street began, or where the front lawn or sidewalks ended because everything was a solid white. The snow blowing toward our house was heavy and moist. It reminded me of angel food cake after it was sliced. I was patiently waiting for it to stop snowing so I could go outside and enjoy sledding.

A little past noon, it stopped as suddenly as it had begun, and it wasn't long before neighbors and others who drove cars, ventured out on the streets. Then the older boys in our family started shoveling a path from the basement door, up around the side-yard to the sidewalk, up the sidewalk and across to the front porch, so we could open the door. In other words, we were truly *snowed in.*

As soon as the cars packed the snow down a little, we could get out our sleds and head for the street. On this particular day, a proud boy from the east side of town brought his handmade bobsled to our street. It was a sight to see, and a gathering of neighbor kids, as well as members of our family, were ready and eager to have their first ride on this magnificent bobsled. It was cold outside, so everyone was bundled up warmly to face the nippy weather.

This super-sized sled would hold ten or twelve kids, while Jim, the owner-driver, sat up in front on a small sled, capable of making quick turns, and which was securely connected by a coupling to the front of the attached, huge sled. There were footboards hanging below this long seat where we placed our feet. By the time the snow was packed enough, it was early afternoon, and Jim was anxious to try out his bobsled. Our home, at 609 West Fifth, was the fourth house down from the top of Fifth Street Hill, and our street was the most popular street in town for sledding. Kids from the east side of town knew this and sometimes came over to join in the fun on our hill.

I was watching them through the window until I could see them lining up to pile on the sled, and then I quickly put on my woolen coat, stocking cap, galoshes, and mittens. I tied a woolen scarf around the neck of my coat, and I was ready. "Hey, wait for me," I shouted, as I ran out the front door. Luckily, I was small enough to be squeezed in, and nobody seemed to mind.

"Okay, you guys, we're ready," shouted Jim, "someone shove off."

The guy on the end shoved us off and jumped back on the sled, and we were moving . . ."Gung-Ho" . . . headed for Second Street . . . the main shopping street in town. "Downtown here we come," we yelled, in unison.

Six blocks down from the top of Fifth was Iowa Avenue, where we would make a quick right. Fifth was steep and slick, and we were gaining momentum. When we reached Iowa Avenue, Jim guided the bobsled in a wide sweep, turning right, and everyone screamed wildly. It was crazy! Drivers pulled their cars over to the side, moving slowly, not believing their eyes. We continued on another three blocks, screaming all the way; but, as we drew closer to Second Street, the street began to level off because this was the downtown shopping area, and the bobsled quickly slowed down to a complete stop. Everyone groaned in unison, knowing we had reached the bottom, and we would have to walk back up to the top of Fifth.

Suddenly, Jim noticed the City Bus had pulled around the corner and had stopped to pick up shoppers. "How lucky can we be," shouted Jim, "you guys give me a hand, and we'll hook the rope to the back of the bus." Everybody cooperated, some pushing, some pulling. The back of the bus had four-inch spikes on the rear bumper to discourage anyone from sitting on it and sneaking a free ride.

"Wow, that's great," said Jim, "just what we need." He quickly hooked the rope over the spikes on the center of the bumper, and putting his forefinger to his lips . . . motioning . . . "Quiet guys . . . jump on"! We didn't need a second invitation, and everyone climbed on.

The bus took off slowly, climbing up Iowa Avenue to Fourth Street, making a left turn and climbing up Fourth, stopping several times to unload passengers. Each time it stopped, the bus passengers observed the bobsled passengers riding on the back, and each time, they saw the bobsled passengers hold their forefingers to their lips, begging them not to give their presence away to the bus driver.

At the top of Fourth was a small neighborhood park, shaped in a circle. The bus driver made a right

turn around the park and then stopped at the next cor-
ner to unload passengers. Jim jumped off the bobsled,
and quickly lifted the rope off the bumper. As the bus
pulled away from the curb, Jim turned to us and or-
dered: "O.K. you guys, everyone off." We knew what
he meant, for there was a steep decline to the bottom,
of Fifth Street, where we would begin the next ride.
It took several of the guys to hold the bobsled back
while we walked as the street was steep. Reaching the
bottom, everyone piled back on the bobsled, and we
headed down the hill again. It was a blast! We were
in for a terrible surprise when we arrived back to the
shopping street, though. Some *party poopers* ruined our
good time. We soon learned that someone must have
called the bus company and registered a complaint, be-
cause the bus driver put a stop to it. He said he couldn't
be held responsible if there was an accident. That was
the end of our hitching free rides behind the bus—our
fun only lasted one time. Jim never came again.

Our hill was always full of kids, mostly because our
family was so large, and we had neighborhood friends
who were also from large families. I have never been
sorry for being part of a large family. Being children
is all about having fun. However, having fun requires
having lots of boys in your midst, because I have learned
that it's always boys who have the most vivid and dar-
ing imaginations.

One day, the guys found a perfectly wonderful place
to build a *hippo*. In case you don't know what that is, I
will explain. Girls run out of enthusiasm when it comes

to shoveling snow, but boys have bigger muscles, and when they get an idea, they never stop until it materializes. They found a small hill two blocks down from where we lived and built their hippo on top of it. The boys packed lots of snow in a heap to create a small knoll on top of this hill. The idea was to ride your sled downhill so you could increase your speed, and when you finally reached the hippo, over you'd fly, free as a bird, and it was fun, because you felt like you were airborne for awhile. However, you had to make a quick turn to the left when you approached this hippo to cross over it. The city dump was just twenty feet beyond this hippo. Country farmers brought their shelled corncobs to this dump. Old, worn-out, junked automobiles ended up at the bottom of this burial ground, and everyone threw their unwanted junk items there, too. It was the city dump! If you weren't careful when you flew over the hippo, you would continue into the dump, which made it even more daring. The idea was to turn your sled quickly before this happened so you didn't end up at the bottom. The problem is explaining this to a six-year-old. My younger sister, Phyllis, found out the hard way. We heard her screaming for help, and someone had to go down and rescue her. Fortunately, she only suffered scratches and bruises, and survived with only bad memories, for luckily, she landed in a heap of corncobs. The rest of us learned to turn our sleds sharply to the right before we reached the edge of the dump.

Tony Smit, the boy who lived next door and to the left of us, came flying down the hill headed for the hippo on his brand-new, bright-red, Radio Flyer, which he got for Christmas, and ran smack into me. Some bigger kid had jumped on his back and put his hands over Tony's eyes, and Tony couldn't see where he was going. The front of his sled had a metal bumper, which stuck out about six inches in front of the turning handles. He was going fast when the bumper hit my leg, but I never felt a thing. The next I knew, I woke up in bed with a broken leg. The doctor had to come to our house to set the bone. He put a plaster of paris splint on it, patted me on the head when I opened my eyes for a second, smiled at me and left. Later, the kids told me I was 'knocked-cold' and they had pulled me home on a sled. Mom threw up her hands in shock, called the doctor, and I became the hit of the neighborhood! Everyone came to see me so they could sign their name on the whitestone bandage. One day the doctor came by to remove the plaster of paris splint, and when I saw the small saw he carried, I thought he was going to saw my leg off, and I started to cry. He patted my head gently and said, "Now, now, young lady, this isn't going to hurt a bit." He proceeded to carefully saw through the plaster cast, while I squinted my eyes in a grimace, not daring to look.

Finally, he said, "You can open your eyes now; I'm through." There, lying neatly on the bed beside my leg was my most treasured memento . . . the cast with all the signatures intact. I knew I would never throw it away! Mama said it smelled to high heaven, because my leg hadn't been washed for weeks, but I didn't care. To me, it was like a beautiful picture, and if I had it my way, I would have hung it on the wall forever. Strangely, one day it disappeared, and I believed one of my jealous kid sisters or brothers took it, but my mother just smiled when I told her my thoughts and said, "Let's all go out in the kitchen, I just baked some Toll House cookies," and I temporarily forgot about the cast. My mother's cookies were great, but I will never really forget about my broken leg and the disappearance of the cast.

Tony Smit played a small romantic part in my life later, when I reached the age of ten. He was about five years older than me. His family originated from Holland, and Tony had beautiful wavy, blond hair and the clearest blue eyes I had ever seen. I never really noticed how handsome he was, until one day at the neighborhood grocery store. When he was through purchasing his groceries, I saw him buy himself a chocolate ice cream cone. I noticed he was kind of hanging around the vegetables by the doorway while I was getting my groceries. As I approached him, he said, "Um-m-m-m, this cone is really great."

"It sure looks good, Tony," I said, but thinking to myself, some kids have all the luck, because we never had money to buy ice cream cones.

"Oh, hey," said Tony, "do you want one? I'll buy you one."

I didn't know what to say. I looked at him, and all I could think of was, *yes,* but I just couldn't say it. I was too shy, and I looked down at the ground, not saying a word.

"Come on," he said, as he headed back to the ice cream counter, "What flavor would you like?"

"Really?" I replied, as I followed him. "I would like chocolate." *Just like his,* I thought. After he purchased my cone, and as we started down the sidewalk towards home, I darted a good glance at him. He was more than a head taller than me, and I really saw him for the first time. I noticed how good looking he was, and I wondered that maybe, because he had bought me a cone, it meant he wanted to be my boyfriend. I was only ten years old, but I suddenly wondered if he thought I was cute. I began to think that maybe I was kind of cute, at least cute enough to buy an ice cream cone for. Looking back, I'll bet he was just trying to make up for breaking my leg that day, while sledding in the snow. Nothing grew from this first experience of getting to know Tony better because he eventually moved away. I later learned that he and his mother were living next door with his grandparents, but it was just a temporary thing. Many years later, when his grandparents had passed on, Tony returned to live in this house. I met his new wife, who was really a lovely woman, and later gave birth to a little girl. Looking back, I remember wishing I could have known him better, married him, and been the mother of this little girl, but I guess it just wasn't meant to be. That's life, I guess!

Ted

My earliest memory of Ted, my oldest brother, born December 13, 1905, Mom's first-born child in her family of nineteen children, when he was 21, was that he was very tall and slim, had black, wavy hair and very dark, kind-eyes. I was four and would run happily down our front sidewalk to meet him when he came home from work.

I also remember that he would swing me up above his head and let me walk upside down on the ceiling of our living room. I trusted him, and knew he would not let me fall. Because he didn't mind spending his time with us and taught us how to have lots of fun, he stands out in my memory now. He loved all eighteen of us younger siblings, and we loved him, too.

Looking back to when I was five years old in 1927, and Ted was 22, I remember how he taught us to make whistles out of the green boughs of young saplings growing in the ravine below our house. Our house, in Mucatine, Iowa, was on top of a hill, and he would take us down to the small creek below, where the young saplings grew, and show us how to choose the perfect size for carving whistles. He cut sections about five inches long with his pocket knife, and then he carved a small notch about an inch from the end, removed the notch, and rubbed the green bark with the dull side of the knife blade until, with just a small twist, the bark would slide easily off the wood. Then, he would carve a little bit of wood from the notched end, replace the green bark so we could blow through that end, and it would make a very high-pitched whistle. We were small children, and he was a grown man, but because it was during the Great Depression, he did things for us to make up for our lack of toys.

When Ted decided to move out of our home to find employment in Chicago, which was about 210 miles from Muscatine, we missed him very much, but, as promised, he did visit us often.

On one of his visits, he took us fishing to South Muscatine where we could catch catfish. He piled a bunch of us in his *Tin Lizzie,* his Ford, two-seater, and off we went on our first great fishing adventure. First he showed us how to bait the hook with worms. This was quite an experience, because we had to dig for the worms, which we never knew lived in our garden Then he showed us how to slide the worm over the hook, which upset us because we felt sorry for the worms. He cut a section of a tree branch, about six inches long, tied a piece of fishing tackle to its center, and on the other end of the line, he attached another six inch section of a branch, on which he had whittled a sharp point. We could string the pointed end of the branch through the gill of the fish and slide the fish down to the end of the string. The first piece of branch kept the fish from escaping. Then we would stick the sharpened branch into the ground at the water's edge and toss the fish back into the water. This would keep the fish fresh while we continued to catch other fish. Ted was a very patient, and a very good, loving brother.

Finally, our lines were full of small catfish, so Ted decided we should pack up and head for home. I was now seven, the oldest of the others, so I sat beside Ted in the front seat. It was beginning to get dark, he quickly started Old Lizzie's motor, and we headed for home. We had just traveled a short distance when I realized he was traveling on the wrong side of the road, and I quickly said, "Ted, do you know you're driving on the wrong side of the road?"

He said, "Oh! Okay," and he steered the car over to the right side of the center line. "I couldn't see the line," he said, "because it's getting a little dark." He drove slowly the rest of the way, and we arrived home safely.

Later when I told Mama of the incident, she said, "Oh, dear. I completely forgot to tell you. He lost the sight in his left eye when he was a young boy, while playing in the creek with his friends. They were throwing spear-like, old, dead, corn stalks that they had pulled out of the ground, at each other. They had dirt clods on one end, because it made the stalks sail further, and he got hit in his left eye which caused him to lose the sight in that eye."

Later, I noticed that Ted's left eye had a glazed look about it, and from that day on, I worried about Ted driving his car home from Chicago, but he always traveled in the daytime and never had a problem. He just wasn't able to drive at night.

I recall another incident when I was about ten, and my sister Jo Ann was about eight. Ted had come home to visit, and had just purchased a new, bright-yellow, 1932 Ford Roadster, the model with a rumble seat in the back. Jo Ann and I were so excited that we wanted to go out and sit in the car. Ted said it was okay, but that we shouldn't touch anything because it could be very dangerous. Jo Ann and I sat in the front seat of the car and the three younger ones climbed in the rumble seat. Ted was in a hurry when he parked the car in front of our house, (for it was facing the wrong direction on our side of the street), and was parked going down hill. The hill was very steep, so he had turned the left front wheel toward the curb and had set the handbrake, thinking it was safely parked.

As the eldest, and in the driver's seat, I put my hands on the steering wheel, pretending to drive. Jo Ann, excited, grabbed the handbrake, and unaware of what she was doing, squeezed the brake lever—releasing it. The car began to move. Fortunately, Ted had turned the wheel to the curb, but the car moved up over the curb, and then rolled slowly across our front lawn. We all started to scream, but that didn't stop the car! At the end of our property, and separating it from our next door neighbor's property, stood a very old, oak tree, but luckily, the trunk of the tree was wide enough to stop the car. We hit it with a loud bang, and we all jumped out of the car in a flash, running, screaming, into the house, hunting for Ted, leaving the front door of our house hanging wide open.

Ted knew something bad had happened, and naturally, he knew it had to do with his car. We were all talking so fast over the top of each other, and he only said, "My, God, what has happened." Without another word, he rushed to the open door, looked out, and saw his car smashed up against the tree, and then, he turned to us.

"Is anyone hurt?" he asked.

"No," I said, "but Ted, are you upset?"

"Don't worry about a thing. The important thing is, no one is hurt. I can fix the car." That was our brother Ted.

We all learned from that day on that we had the most wonderful brother anyone could have, and that we all loved him very much. Mamma and Papa were not at home at the time and Ted decided not to tell them about the incident, thinking it would just upset them. Ted moved his car back to the curb, parking it correctly, going uphill, with the back of the right front wheel angled to the curb, and warned us never to get in it again. Luckily, he only had to replace the front bumper, but what would have happened if the tree hadn't been there?

We lost Ted, our oldest brother, at the age of forty-nine. He died in his sleep from a fatal heart attack following dental surgery. The dentist had given him a sedative for the removal of all of his teeth, in preparation for false teeth. A younger brother took him home and put him to bed, but Ted later had a heart attack while asleep, and never woke up. The dentist claimed he wasn't aware that Ted's heart was weak or he wouldn't have given him the sedative.

Ted's heart may have been too weak for a sedative, nevertheless, I know, as do many others, that his heart was full of love. I will always treasure the memories of the brother who spent time with us, taught us so much, and whom we all loved in return.

My Greek Vacation

It was the summer of 1982. I had been invited to join a tour group with members of my voice class at Golden West College, Huntington Beach, California. This was a time in my life when I really needed something to add excitement to my life, and I thought, *why not?* I had just gone through a very disturbing time obtaining a divorce from a mentally and physically abusive husband, and was not coping very well with the adjustment. I really needed a change, something to help me forget about the past and make a new start. This was the perfect time in my life to get away; especially a cruise.

I had never been on a cruise, and this would be a special vacation, touring the Greek Islands, Egypt, Israel, Turkey and Cyprus. We would see many things I had often wondered about, especially in the Holy Land. Our ship, the MTS ORION, would cruise the blue Aegean, and we would be enjoying the usual fare, with meals on board, swimming in the deck pool, or just lulling in the desk chairs or sunbathing. I finally made up my mind. I was happy to accept the invitation. I needed it!

We met at the Los Angeles Airport on August 17th, and we boarded a Trans World Airlines flight heading across the ocean in the direction of Athens, Greece. We arrived there on August 18th, met our tour guide who assisted us through Customs, and then headed toward our hotel, the Parthenon. We were shown our rooms, and then herded back to the lounge for a welcome cocktail party, followed by a lovely dinner. This was at 6:00 P.M. on the second day of our journey. The muscles in my back and neck began to relax, and I realized what it was like to forget my troubles and have fun.

The following day began at 6:00 A.M. We ate our breakfast and, then at 6:30, we departed on a tour bus through the City of Athens. After a scenic drive, passing by the Tomb of the Unknown Soldier, Parliament, the Presidential Palace, and the National Archaeological Museum, we headed in the direction of the Acropolis. One member of our tour bus was in a wheelchair, and before we began the climb up the long stone stairway to the top of the hill to see the ruins of the Acropolis, I told him that I would look for him when we came back down so he wouldn't be left behind when we boarded the bus to return to the hotel. This turned out to be a big mistake!

After our tour through the ruins of the Acropolis, I began to wish I had studied a little about the history of this country before making the trip. We did see some films in preparation, but if it were not for the literature I reviewed when I returned home, I discovered I was completely ignorant about Greece. Never take a tour without a thorough study!

When we began to descend the stairs, as I had promised, I hurried ahead of my group to look for the gentleman in the wheelchair. He was nowhere to be found. I finally gave up because the rest of the group was impatient to return to the hotel, so I went back to the foot of the steps and discovered they had left me. Now, where was the bus? To my dismay, I discovered there were three paths leading out from the steps. There was nothing I could do but pick one and hope it led back to the bus. The first two were disappointments, and I became frantic on the third path, as I ran down in the direction of the street. When I got there, there was no bus! I saw an officer directing traffic in the center of the street, and I ran to him. "Have you seen my bus?" I asked.

"Oh, yes, Madam," he said, "it left at least ten minutes ago."

I couldn't believe my ears. My group left without me! I asked the officer for help. He hailed a passing taxi, and he told me the taxi would take me back to my hotel. The problem was, the taxi driver was Greek and did not speak fluent English, and because I was upset, my mind blanked out, and I had a difficulty recalling the name of the hotel. Finally remembering, we headed for the Parthenon. Unfortunately, he was new on the job and was just becoming familiar with places in the city. Each time he stopped the taxi, it was not my hotel. There were several businesses and even cocktail bars by the same name. About an hour later, he finally found the hotel. While traveling, I explained that because my group had left me behind, I was very upset, and I apologized for displaying it. When we arrived, he walked me to the door, and opened it because he could see how distressed I really was with my group.

As I entered the hotel, I could see them in the bar, sitting around having cocktails. Strangely, the man in the wheelchair was not at the hotel, and I later learned he had joined the tour on his own. I had previously told my driver that in the evening, we were to go on a tour of Athens by night. It was to start at the "Top-of-the-Hill" with a sound and light presentation, followed by a dinner and a floor show with bouzouki music at a typical *Plaka taverna,* returning to the hotel after midnight.

At the door, I thanked him for his trouble, and asked him how much I owed him. He refused my fare, and quickly introduced himself: "My name is Georgi Slakia," he said, and then, he asked me if he could be my escort for the evening's festivities. He was a good-looking man, but with an unattractive beard. He was probably somewhere in his forties, and I was now sixty, although people usually gave me a twenty-year-leeway, so I was flattered at his invitation. I asked him if he knew where the "Top of the Hill" was, and he said he did. So, I decided, why not? I'd show my group I didn't need them for my fun, so I accepted, and he said he would pick me up in about two hours. I went to my room to lie down for a little rest, and then took a quick shower and dressed. I had told my group that I wouldn't be going with them, because I would have an escort, and they were very surprised. I introduced them to him, and then told my new friend, Georgi, that we were to meet in the lounge at 7:00 p.m. for our evening of fun.

My escort arrived at seven o'clock sharp. At first, I didn't recognize him, then was completely shocked by his appearance. He was dressed in a white suit, his beard was newly coifed, and he entered the lounge where I was waiting. He was so handsome! I thought we would be traveling on the bus, but he insisted that he drive me in his taxi, so we left the group standing there, and they were, needless to say, as shocked as I was stunned at his appearance.

My escort led me to his taxi, opened the door, and we drove off. After we had traveled a mile or so, he suddenly said, "Yes, this is the place." He parked the car, opened my door, and led me to an elevator door. He pressed a button, the door opened, and he escorted me into the elevator.

"Where are we going?" I questioned.

"Up," he said, "to the Top of The Hill." The elevator climbed upwards, until we reached the eighteenth floor, the doors opened and I stepped out and could see that we were on the top of the building. The floor was covered with luxurious carpeting and dining tables draped in white tablecloths, with fancy wrought-iron chairs surrounding them. The area was fully protected from the elements with a sheltering roof, and windows extending from the roof to a three-foot wall, which surrounded the entire floor.

It was clear to me that the Top of The Hill was a restaurant. I walked over to the wall and looking through the window could see the spectacular view of the city of Athens beyond. In the far distance, I saw a gathering of bright lights on a hilltop, and I said, "I wonder what's going on over there?"

"Oh," he said, "that's the Acropolis."

"Wait a minute," I exclaimed, "that's where I think my group is. They're not here, and I think we are in the wrong place. Don't tell me it's happened again. If they are not here in another half hour, I want to go over there."

They never showed up, but I was starved, and finally, in resignation, I said, "Well, I guess we should have dinner. They're not coming. We're on the wrong Top of The Hill." I was beginning to see why Athens was a tourist city! Before you left, you visited the whole city!

"I'm so sorry," he said, "but don't worry, we'll have some fun. I'll take you to a few of the places I like." (His English was *broken,* but I was soon able to decipher his meaning.)

We ate our dinner, and very shortly headed back down in the elevator. Georgi took me to see Athens at night, and I discovered it is a very lively city. The people there are very gracious and friendly. We eventually stopped at a very popular cocktail bar where a Greek wedding was taking place. The maitre d' led us to a table where we could see the wedding party. A very long table was placed opposite the entrance, and the guests of the wedding party were seated around the table. We ordered Pallini, a white wine, which Georgi said was the best Greek wine, and when it was delivered, the waiter told us the bride and groom would be honored if we would join their group. I was flattered to be invited, and said, "Oh, I would like that." We walked over and were seated. Soon, the wedding ceremony began. Because it was a Greek wedding, and, as was the custom, the couple completed the ceremony by breaking their champagne glasses, throwing them on the floor and stomping on them, and we then formed a circle around the bridal couple, encircling our arms around each other, and we all joined in a traditional dance around the bride and groom, while the sounds of orchestrated Greek wedding music filled the room. I was thoroughly delighted at being allowed to share in this part of the Greek culture. When we left, I felt like I couldn't have had a more perfect evening. We returned to the Parthenon Hotel, and I thanked my escort for his graciousness. We had previously discussed my busy travel schedule, and we knew this was probably the only time we would see each other. We hugged goodbye, and I felt truly blessed to have met my new friend, Georgi.

After he left, I noticed my group was there ahead of me again having cocktails, and I could tell they were full of envy and questions about my date as I must have been glowing with happiness. I told them all goodnight and left them with their curiosity unsatisfied as to the reason why I hadn't joined them. That was my secret!

We left Athens on the eighth day of our tour. It was to be a fifteen-day experience, and somehow, I felt the rest could not compare with this wonderful beginning. However, I was soon to discover it was just a wonderful beginning. I had a marvelous time throughout my trip and took lots of pictures in Egypt, Israel, Turkey and Cyprus. Each country gave me memories that are still with me. I never dreamed I would ever experience such things in my lifetime. I arrived home relaxed and satisfied, knowing it was just what I needed to start my new life.

Richard Wrate

Well, yes, we write memoirs, political arguments, scientific papers for laypeople, and short stories and novels. But we also pen documentaries—or at least Dick Wrate does. If it were a video rather than a writing workshop, Dick could rival Ken Burns. Interestingly, the first of his work that any of us saw was a moving and mystic nature story, a piece of writing in a genre of its own. I think I sense echoes of that first piece in the bear story that follows.

—W.R.W.

FOREWORD

My story, Beauty in the Beast, happened during the fall seasons of 2000 and 2001. Presently in 2007, in California where I live and Colorado where I play, attention is once more focused on the plight of the black bear. A widespread drought is affecting all wildlife right where it hurts the most—their stomach. Once more, the acorn crop in the mountains of Colorado is decimated by an early frost. In Big Bear and the Tahoe area, berries are shriveling on the vine. Lean bruins are putting hibernation on hold to better garner a full stomach.

Clashes between humans and bears in both the Rockies and the Sierras are at an all time high. In order to fill their stomach, the ursine population is entering homes and dining in someone's kitchen. Black Bears are facing a test of survival. For many of us who love the animals of the forest, we must listen to the bear's plight and act on their behalf.

Beauty in the Beast

The August 31, 2000, issue of the *Aspen Times*, reads:

LIFE GETS EVEN TOUGHER FOR THE BEAR POPULATION (*MY SUMMARY*)

In the year 2000, bears' natural foods, such as berries and acorns suffered ruin from an early freeze. Road kill was at an all time high. The Colorado Department of Wildlife (DOW) put down more nuisance bears than any year in memory. To make bruin life more unbearable, bear hunting began September 1st, and continued throughout the month. If every hunter killed one bear and every *nuisance* bear was put down, then add the high mortality on the highways, there would be no bears left in Colorado. I ask, why does the state continue to allow hunting, especially under these adverse conditions? Not only do bears have to run and hide from hunters, they are

forced by nature to be up and about twenty
hours a day foraging for adequate fattening
food in order to sustain a fast throughout
their long hibernation.(John Colson, *Aspen
Times, 7 September 2000*)

DOW: Bruins Don't Need Help

An unknown but vocal number of Aspenites want local
governments to take steps to feed the starving bears
who recently have been rampaging through town re-
cently.

Aspen and the upper Roaring Fork Valley have been
dealing with an unprecedented number of bear sight-
ings and bear-human interactions since the beginning
of summer.

The cause of this invasion, according to Colorado
Division of Wildlife (DOW) experts, is a lack of the
bear's natural food sources in the high country com-
bined with a growing familiarity with and loss of fear of
humans. Residents, well aware of the bear's plight, have
concluded that the best way to help the bears and end
the intrusions into neighborhoods and homes would be
for the government to mount a feeding program.

"A fed bear is a happier, more respectful bear," main-
tained local real estate broker Chris Leverich, in a letter
to Colorado legislator Russell George of Rifle. "If the
DOW allowed volunteers to take food to designated
remote locations, within a matter of weeks, many bears
would be drawn out of the urban areas, our back yards,

and our kitchens. If the bears were fed now, they'd have a better chance to go into the winter healthy."

The following is taken from a September 8, 2000, article in the *Aspen Times*.

It's Just This Simple: Leave the Bears Alone, Please

Some locals, saddened by the likely outcome that many cubs and yearlings will starve in their dens this winter, believe it is our duty to dump food in the backcountry where the bears can find it. The problem is that, even if we could somehow manage to provide them with enough food to do any good (a questionable concept), this would only make matters worse. Bears, already habituated to humans and used to raiding our garbage for their sustenance, would only become more dependent on us. Their life cycles would suffer from our interference.

The following is a September 22, 2000, article in the *Aspen Times* by Scott Condon

Bear-Feeding Backer Unswayed

The man who helped spark debate about feeding beleaguered bears this summer said he hasn't heard any criticism that's swayed his opinion.

Aspenite Chris Leverich, wrote a letter to new DOW director Russell George, who he said is a friend, earlier this month suggesting that food be provided to bears in remote sites, far from towns like Aspen. The feeding was proposed as a way to keep the bears from rummaging around town looking for food. Leverich said he doesn't think bear feeding should be undertaken unless there's an emergency, like this year's severe shortage in food supply. Wildlife officials have estimated that half the bear cubs won't survive the winter because of a lack of berries and acorns this summer and fall. In addition, a record number of bears have been intentionally killed in Colorado for being so-called nuisances . . .

The idea gained regional and even national attention from media reporting on Colorado's and Aspen's problems with hungry bruins. The plan has produced lively debate, pro and con, in letters to local newspapers.

The charm and natural beauty I love about Aspen took a back seat to brother bears' food crisis. To my knowledge, not one local had publicly admitted feeding bears. "Feeding bears is a punishable crime," announced the Colorado Department of Wildlife.

With timidity aside, I crossed that line on September 26, 2000. A news headline, ably written by Allyn Harvey, was released in the *Aspen Times*.

Man Says, "He Feeds Bruins"

> A part-time Aspen resident admitted yesterday that he is feeding the bears, and he vowed to keep it up as long as he can, even if it is against the law. Richard Wrate, who has been visiting Aspen since 1962, said he has been trucking 50-pound bags of Cobb—a mix of corn, oat, barley and molasses mix ranchers and farmers feed to livestock—into the backcountry and leaving it out for the bears. Over the last two weeks, Wrate estimates that he's left 1,000 pounds of the stuff at twelve sites around the upper valley.

Comment: If Cobb can fatten up livestock and is healthy for horses, why not beef-up undernourished bears with a natural food of choice. One sniff of molasses and the bear population will be hooked.

[Todd] Malmsbury [of the Colorado DOW] said, "He's interfering with nature. We know that in good years wildlife population increases, and in bad years the population declines, but he's stepping in at a time when the overall population is in no danger of starvation."

Comment: Okay, so Malmsbury feels bears should move to Minnesota or Upper Michigan where acorns are plentiful this year. I prefer to save bears from starvation right here in the valley.

[Malmsbury] "At first, the bags of food Wrate left in the upper Roaring Fork River and Castle Creek valleys went untouched, except maybe by a few birds and deer who happened by. But once Wrate added apples and honey to the mix, local ursines took notice. He says he's sure the food is going to the bears because of the way the bags have been shredded." . . .

Wrate said there is no longer a need to add honey, which makes the whole effort a lot more affordable. A 50-pound bag of Cobb goes for $6.22, according to a saleswomen at the Roaring Fork Valley Co-op in Carbondale.

Comment: Hungry bears, when searching for food, frequent rivers and streams. Just the place to smear honey on unopened bags of Cobb. Success came when I found bear tracks and observed bruins clawing open the bags. Not wanting to be called a litterbug, I collected each shredded bag.

Most felt the feeding of bears necessary during their time of lack; however, one guy at the Carbondale co-op told me: "I can't sell Cobb to you. It's not for bears, ya know."

My evenings were spent at the Aspen Public Library studying behavior of the beautiful beast. Mother bearman, Ben Kilham, became my mentor. He authored *Among the Bears*, which I read from cover to cover. I discovered what it's like to live the life of a bear. *Sacred Paw* is a classic when it comes to bear behavior. Dozens of other books on bruins helped me to better understand this giant of the forest.

September 26, 2000, the *Aspen Times* continued:

> The 69-year-old California resident said he is perfectly aware of the warnings and pronouncements issued by state and local wildlife experts. "I can understand their arguments, but this is an exceptional year." Wrate said.
>
> In today's letter to the editor, Wrate urged people who are concerned about the well-being of the bears to begin their own feeding programs. "In the last few days we have seen that winter is fast approaching. Those who are able should start a grassroots project of feeding bears," he writes. "All of us can write or call the Department of Wildlife. Make a fuss! By coming into town— the bears did."

Comment: My letter to the editor was a smashing success. Several dozen callers wanted to give of their time and money. I could not accept their contributions; however, when I wasn't allowed to purchase more Cobb, several locals bought the Cobb for me.

Malmsbury also pointed out that each bear requires a square mile of habitat, so feeding stations like the ones established by Wrate probably aren't helping very many bears.

Comment: Okay, Mr. Malmsbury, tell your story to the bears I helped.

Next morning, a bomb was delivered with the *Aspen Times* newspaper—a blaring headline:

DOW Investigates Bear Feeder

Aspen Times, September 27, 2000.
By Allyn Harvey.

"There could be more than one ticket in this case," said the DOW's Todd Malmsbury. "It's $68.00 per ticket, which isn't a lot, but he could potentially be fined, for every single instance he placed food out for the bears." . . .

Wrate said he was motivated to action after hearing of a motherless cub in Redstone that was wandering through town begging for food . . .

"That probably got me going more than anything else"

Comment: Yes, seeing to the needs of a motherless cub can be a real motivational force. After the cub's attendance at a lawn wedding at the Redstone Inn, I heard he stole a blueberry pie from the Inn's kitchen. The youngster soon became known as the Blueberry Bear of Redstone. Each unlocked pantry was an open invitation to a full stomach. Redstones population of 92 had risen to 93. I did want to meet the newest resident; but our meeting was never to be. One day while feeding bears outside the Redstone limits, I read a copy of the *Aspen Times*. A startling letter to the editor caught my attention, I read the first line: CUB KILLER. In shock I read the article. Blueberry Bear was dead.

Anne Grigutis' letter on CUB KILLER:

Dear Editor:

To the killer of our little cub.

What brave man killed our poor, defenseless little cub? How proud you must be to have killed the cub that practically everyone in Redstone had taken to its heart.

I understand that you used a bow and arrow. This cub was so tame and trusting that it must have been easy, or did you tie him to a tree and then do it? A man with no scruples could.

One day the little cub came to my kitchen window, which was open, and we looked closely at one another. I asked him what he was doing trying to get in my kitchen. He looked at me, hung his head and walked off the deck. But he looked back over his shoulder once as though he wanted me to know that he wasn't so bad.

I know things can change when bears are fully grown, but couldn't you have given him a chance? Hibernation is not far off and he may have survived. You can't imagine the delight of everyone who saw the cub and took photos. He was so unconcerned, and went walking along, minding his own business. He was no threat to anyone.

I have lived in Redstone for 11 years, and this is the first bear I have ever seen. People still come into my shop and ask for him, but unfortunately our little cub with the two red earrings is gone, and I must say that, as an animal lover, I grieve.

Did it ever occur to you that it is illegal to kill a cub? My hope is that you will be caught and punished.

Anne Grigutis. Redstone, owner of Trayde Castle of hand made porcelain dolls.

I hurried to Anne's shop. I found her sincere and charming. Tearfully, she offered stories and pictures of Blueberry; spending over an hour telling me about the only bear she ever knew.

One touching incident occurred when Anne left a peach pie to cool on her windowsill. When a hairy arm reached up to take the pie, she hollered: "STOP!" The rascal ran. He did not get her pie, and, strangely enough, that saddened Anne. Before nightfall, she left on her porch four ripe peaches along with peach peelings and pits. Next morning she found all the peaches and peelings eaten, with each bit of peach flesh removed from the pit. Anne remembered how this bear had overturned many a Redstone trashcan, but here on her back porch every pit had been neatly assembled in a pile. From then on, she left scraps of food she thought a bear might like. So did her neighbors. Within a few days, the garbage cans in Redstone were all left upright, The little bruin's table manners had definitely improved.

I always make it a rule to visit Redstone when vacationing in Aspen. I should have jumped in my van when hearing about the orphan cub. Had I done so, a life lost might have been spared. Even now, while writing this story, I feel guilty. Earlier, I put in a call to Nanci Limbach, at the Animal Rehabilitation Center, hoping she might help our orphan find a den for the winter. She knew of Redstone's new resident and she also knew that since he was a yearling, the Department of Wildlife would not allow the transfer. He wore two red rings clipped to one ear, meaning he had been twice removed from an unknown community, which made him a two-time loser. I left Redstone with many treasured memories of our beloved Blueberry Bear. I was now more dedicated then ever to feeding our starving neighbors.

Continuation of September 27, DOW Investigates Bear Feeder:

[Malmsbury] "Not only will his actions—which are illegal, inappropriate and ineffective—impact the bears, they'll impact deer and other wildlife as well," he said. "He's taking the wild out of wildlife by disrupting the natural process."

Wrate has been breaking a law that makes it a misdemeanor to intentionally feed big game. The $68.00 ticket can be applied to every sack of Cobb that Wrate has dropped in the backcountry. As of Tuesday, Wrate says he has dropped 1,000 pounds, or 20 sacks, adding up to a potential fine of $1,360. Although Wrate could no be reached for comment for this story, he did vow on Tuesday to continue feeding bears.

Comment: Mr. Malmsbury, I fed bears until leaving for California on October 3, 2000. I willingly take blame for placing 226 bags of Cobb and since you are fining me $68.00 a bag, your figures should show $15,368 owed to the Department of Wildlife. However, since it is now October 2007, I feel the statue of limitations has expired.

Wrate says he's heard that other people are doing the same thing he is, but wasn't able to name any of them.

Comment: I'm no snitch. Dozens called on how they might help. Apart from Malmsbury's criticism, only two negative responses were received. I did have calls from several horse owners who said the co-op was out of Cobb because of large purchases for bears. I volunteered to buy a supply for horses further down valley.

The next day, September 28th, I drove my wife Helen to the Aspen airport. I had kept the DOW Investigates Bear Feeder article from her. With a disappointing fall color showing, and only two days since the knowledge of my feeding bears had become widespread, she was ready to return to the sanctuary of our California home. Had she read the DOW investigation of the local bear feeder, I fear she would have expected jail time for her husband.

Prior to Helen's departure, I became involved in the life of another orphaned cub. While trying to escape from a large male bear, his mother attempted to climb an electric pole in the Buttermilk Ski area. She was electrocuted and the cub we called Buttermilk, scared and alone, hid in a strand of trees between two ski runs.

Several days later, while returning to Aspen, after feeding bears down valley, I decided to stop at the Buttermilk Fruit Stand. I wanted to purchase seconds for bears, and to ask the vendor if the motherless cub had been seen recently. "Only ten minutes ago I caught that rascal in the back of the truck eating my best apples. I chased him up the slope. I'll bet he's still around."

Walking towards the vendor's truck, I thought: That's my winter ski run. If he's still here in December, I better loan him my skis. As I surveyed the groomed incline, now summer green, I saw a small dark object rapidly moving toward a strand of trees.

"It's him!" I exclaimed.

I dashed up the hill and saw the cub disappearing in the dark thicket. I explored the dense brush, but found only bits of apple core. I returned to the fruit vendor who contributed twelve spotted apples. Having promised not to feed bears inside Aspen, I inquired: "Aren't we outside the city limits of Aspen?"

"Sure are, better than a mile."

For Buttermilk's supper I left twelve apples, along with a bag of vegetables and more than ten pounds of Cobb.

That night I dreamed of a little cub, less than a year old, who recently lost his mother. When morning came, I called Nanci Limbach at the animal rehabilitation center. "Nanci, I would like to deliver to you one orphan cub. There's an adult black bear after this cub and you know how territorial they can be."

"Can't do, Richard, without Department of Wildlife authority. If the animal had been injured, that would be a different story." Buttermilk, a yearling, would remain my charge. After Helen left, I continued to feed him and other hungry bears. Ample Cobb was available, but time was running out. It was October 1st, and I had promised Helen I would leave on the 3rd. She wanted me home—while the DOW simply wanted me . . .

Lorraine, a chiropractor whose office was in Glenwood Springs, took an active interest in Buttermilk and our plan to feed starving bears. She sincerely hoped we find a home for our orphaned cub.

The day I was to leave, I received a call from Fox News. They wanted my story on feeding Buttermilk. Good, I thought, this would further our cause in helping bears in crisis.

"Wonder of wonders," exclaimed Lorraine, "a dream come true. With exposure on Fox News, the bear's plight will be nationally released."

The shoot had been scheduled for October 7th. It would be impossible for me to be there. I had made a promise to my wife. I would keep that promise. Lorraine gladly agreed to take my place.

"What a grand way to publicize the bears plight," she said, "Buttermilk will become a symbol of hope for all bears."

"Lorraine, you know I can't be there. I want you to tell our story."

"Of course. Maybe your leaving is for the best. Malmsbury can't chase you to California."

On October 2nd, I got a call from a reporter with the *Denver Post*. They had heard about Fox News's forthcoming coverage of Buttermilk and wanted listeners in the Denver area to know about my feeding bruins. I told the reporter what I knew and gave him Lorraine's phone number, and asked him, "Please don't mention my leaving Aspen."

He readily agreed, and asked for my California phone number and e-mail address. He said their radio affiliate talk show host wanted to do their October 10th program on the present condition of Colorado bears. Todd Malmsbury of DOW, would represent one side of the issue, with me taking the adversarial position.

"We will arrange a three way telephone hook-up," said the reporter.

On my arrival home, I called the radio station. A thirty-minute slot had been set for the show. Early on the 10th, the station called to brief me on protocol. I was told to speak my mind without reservation. I further learned Malmsbury had declined to participate. No matter, I thought, everyone knew of the DOW position. My point could still get across. I'm certain 8,000 bears will applaud my message.

I ended the telephone broadcast with these words: "Thank you, Denver, for listening to my message on this year's food crisis in the bear population. If you wish to help motherless or injured bears, please call

Nanci Limbach at the Pauline S. Schneegas Wildlife Foundation. Nanci presently has 19 bears in her compound, awaiting placement in prepared dens."

Lorraines's attempt to feed Buttermilk Bear was shown as planned on Fox News; however, the cub did not show. Instead, a mammoth black bear took all the bows and every bit of the prepared food. He seemed to enjoy the limelight.

There was no sign of Buttermilk for the remainder of 2000. Winter skiing brought me near his favorite feeding ground. While traversing the slope where Buttermilk had been fed, I tried to imagine him sleeping within a snow-covered thicket nearby.

Early one fall morning, October the 22nd, 2001, I again drove to Aspen. I was alone. Helen had agreed to my spending solitary time with the smaller animals of the forest. Without compromise, she had demanded there be no bear business this season.

Buttermilk Returns?

Looking through the eyes of sleep, I peered out the condo window. The sun blinded my view to the purity of the blue Colorado Sky. For ten days I had been feeding my little fur and feather friends, hoping to write their story.

Yesterday I had prepared a grand feeding for the little folk of the forest. Something for all, but none for bears. This year I had promised my wife Helen I would refrain from feeding the bruin population. Last year each bear I fed thanked me, but the Colorado DOW did not.

Even with the bright sunshine, there was a chill in the air. My loaded van had 20 pounds of overripe grapes. There were also sundry boxes of strawberries and red raspberries, three melons and a bunch of black-skinned bananas, all given by the market as not salable, but a sure treat for birds and other denizens of the forest. In addition, I packed two 25-pound bags of black oil-type sunflower seeds, a favorite fall feeding for squirrels and chipmunks. There was also a sack of critter crunch to be enjoyed by martin and fox. Warmly dressed, armed with a disposable camera, and with enough food to last until dinner, I locked the condo door, and glanced over the balcony railing toward my well-stocked Grand Caravan.

I was stunned! Mounds of scattered bird and sunflower seeds appeared to the right and left of my car. On closer inspection, I found one grape left in a box that only yesterday held 20 pounds. Both side windows had been broken. Glass fragments mixed with birdseed lay scattered about the parking lot. A bear was afoot. Last year I had given food in an attempt to fend off a bruin's insatiable hunger, and look what had happened to me. There was one unopened bag of sunflower seeds, and one open can of almonds, evidently spilled by the bear and scattered beyond his reach.

While cleaning up the mess, I tried to think like a bear in hopes of learning the mystery behind the second broken window, and to focus on a time when the thief would once more appear. I could forgive a bruin stealing food necessary for his survival. Could it be possible he was the orphan cub I fed last summer; but breaking two windows in my Dodge Van? Unforgivable.

I knew he would return the following night, but when? Even if he was Buttermilk, this bruin had a lot of explaining to do. Come on, bear man, think. If I were a hungry bear, what time would I drop in on Mr. Richard? Okay, the next morning stroll for this bear will likely be 4:15 a.m. Throughout the night I dreamed of Buttermilk and how large he had grown. At 4:14, the dream was shattered. Dressed in pajamas and holding a disposable camera, I rushed down the steps in time to see a black bear's bottom protruding from the van's broken side window. He struggled from the small opening and stood up, facing me. His bulk overwhelmed my confidence. I wasn't scared—I was terrified. My pajama pants slipped down to my ankles and I dropped my camera—the camera flash startled brother bear. He lumbered off, without a bite to eat.

I had told a neighbor of my bear encounter, and within a day, it reached the ears of a reporter from the *Aspen Times*. Immediately, Naomi Havlen called for a full report. She said the *Times* had a thick file on me. She held my intruder accountable for the break-in. I pleaded with her not to print the story until my bear was safely lodged in his winter den. "I don't want any harm to come to him. I'm sure you've heard the Department of Wildlife's expression: 'A fed bear is a dead bear.'"

"Look what this bear did to you," she said. "Last year you probably fed this same bear at Buttermilk Mountain and now he rewards you with $1,200 in damages to your van. If that bear returns one more time, he'll be in big trouble with the DOW." I should have known that timely news is rushed to print, faster than any bear hurried to eat Cobb. The following article ripped across the *Aspen Times* headlines:

> Irony That's Hardly Bearable—Man Who Fed Bears Last Summer Has One Break Into His Vehicle
>
> By Naomi Havlen, *Aspen Times* Staff Writer
>
> A man intent on feeding bears illegally last summer had a bruin break into his food-packed car earlier this week in Aspen.
>
> Richard Wrate, who lives in Newport Beach, CA, but visits Aspen several times a year, caused a controversy last year when he spent upwards of $3,000 feeding hungry bears affected by a natural food shortage. . . .
>
> He held off on feeding bears this year, but did buy a large supply of grains to feed birds and chipmunks. Unfortunately, this was the supply Wrate left in his car on Monday evening that wound up in ursine paws . . .
>
> "There is a certain irony in the fact that someone who admitted to feeding the bears illegally would this year be on the receiv-

ing end of hungry bruins right in Aspen," said Todd Malmsbury, spokesman for the Colorado Division of Wildlife. Malmsbury was one of the loudest opponents of Wrate's bear feeding plan last year. "Feeding bears is illegal and inappropriate," he said. "It's bad for the bears, and it's bad for people who live around bears. It only creates more problems rather than solving problems."

Malmsbury said food left by humans for bears even in remote areas can be associated with people through smell. The food attracts the bears, and they begin to depend on it because it's easy to obtain, he said.

But during the summer of 2000, when an early summer freeze severely reduced the natural food supply for bears, the local bruins were routinely cruising alley ways and back yards for sustenance. Wrate said he didn't see the harm in supplying food for bears deep in the wilderness during the time of crisis. "A fed bear has a better disposition than a hungry one," he said. He also said that if bears were smart enough to know where the bags of food were coming from, "they would have taken over Aspen by now." . . .

"It's unfortunate that his car was damaged, but it's even more unfortunate that the bears learned that irresponsible humans can be an excellent source of food." Malmsbury said. Wrate could have been subject to fines in excess of $1,000 for his illegal activities last year, but Wrate had left town before he could be charged . . .

I assumed Buttermilk Bear would make one more appearance. I had to warn him of impending danger. I had heard of Bear-Be-Gone, but was told that ammonia worked just as well. I took one whiff and was certain my bear would keep a safe distance. I thought better than to drench the car with ammonia; so I doused each tire with the stuff. All edibles had been removed, not a single sunflower seed remained. Snow had begun to fall. Lazy flakes first melted then decorated my Dodge van with crystal symmetry. From the local hardware, I purchased a blue tarp, which I draped securely over both broken windows. I weighted down the 12 by 20 foot wrap with fireplace logs. More logs were placed encircling the rear, which made my van appear to be wearing a blue bonnet. Until the window glass arrived, ammonia would mask any enticing leftover smells. No bear, with a sense of smell 50 times that of humans, would visit me tonight.

At precisely 12:15 am., I awoke with a start. Could it be the bruin had returned in spite of my precautions? With a camera, and a safety pin holding up my pajamas, I ventured to the balcony. There he was, peering at the blue tarp where the shattered window had been. He took no notice of me, aware only of the blue bonnet covering his lunch bucket. Lights in the parking lot enlarged a million snowflakes, show-casing a perfect picture. Was there time for a shot? Suddenly, from below, I heard loud huffing and puffing. His body stiffened. With extended claws, he caught the blue tarp, pulling it and the logs down with a thud. Even from the balcony, I could smell the ammonia. I shuddered to think what would happen next. The bear's attention was now riveted on the left rear tire. His paw struck hard, creating a loud hissing sound deep into the night.

My dander was up. This bear had broken two windows and now flattened a tire. Buttermilk would never do that, or would he? Without regard for my safety, I thought only of sending that big puffball a message. I hurried down the steps to confront my nemesis. Less than six feet apart, two bodies froze. We started down one another in icy silence. Might eye-to-eye contact show disrespect? I was filled with intense fear, yet, there were questions to be answered. "Are you my friend Buttermilk? Why did you break the second window?"

Faintly, from the mind of a bear, I sensed the answer. I'm here because of you. I've grown too large to get hold of food, lying out of reach, beyond the first broken window.

However brash, my thoughtful bear was determined only to fill his belly. This I could forgive. As the snow softly descended . . . each of us found mutual respect and gained understanding. I forgave brother bear for crippling my van, as he forgave me for replacing his meal with ammonia.

Which one of us was any less in forgiving? Two individuals bonded as friends, magically joined, in the swirling flakes of snow. I do not know how long we stood peering at one another, but long enough for white bands of snowflakes to cluster about each other's brow.

For his safety, I wanted him to go, and so he did. As he retreated, I was able to snap a picture of my friend as he slowly lumbered off for a five-month slumber in his den.

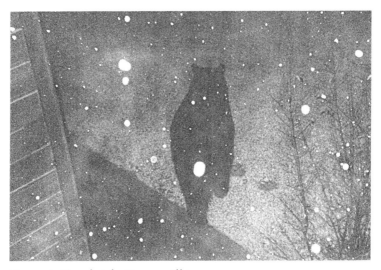

Figure 1. Goodnight Buttermilk!

Contributors

Eddie Hasson (1924-2008) was a California native. He grew up and attended school in Los Angeles graduating from Manual Arts High School in 1943. During World War II, he spent over three years in the Navy as a torpedo man in the submarine service. After the war, he attended George Pepperdine College on the G.I. Bill, and did graduate work at U.S.C. He spent 34 years with the Long Beach Unified School District, teaching Physical Education and Health. He also coached boys gymnastics at Long Beach Polytechnic High School and Long Beach City College.

Mary Ann Huisken (b. 1946) grew up in Downey, California. She graduated in 1968 from Long Beach State College and married her husband Jerry in 1972. She had one child and gained three stepchildren from a later marriage. Though blessed to have lived a life of luxury and be a homemaker, she never forgot the satisfaction she felt from working hard with her cousins and grandparents on their farm in the Midwest. Mary Ann wrote a feature section for *Parents & Kids Magazine,* created a newsletter for her church, and has researched and published numerous family history books. She also did a historical cartoon booklet of an Army Air Force

B-17 crew that was shot down during WWII, and in 1993, did a comprehensive historical book of a nursing school for her mother's fiftieth nursing reunion.

Paul Sammy Larkin (b. 1932) spent his childhood in Springfield, Missouri; his home during his teen years was in Amory, Mississippi, but he spent the months of the school year at a parochial boys school in Arkansas. In 1950, he entered the Trappist Monastery in Gethsemani, Kentucky, as a lay brother. In 1955, he was one of the Trappist brothers who founded a monastery near Vina, California. In 1963, he left the religious order, came to southern California, where he became a real estate broker, and ultimately married. He and his wife, Patricia, reside in Huntington Beach, where she works as a speech pathologist.

Marjory Bong-Ray Liu (b. 1923) is from Nanking, China, and during her first twenty-six years, experienced four internecine conflicts within China, and World War II. She has lived in and traveled over, much of the globe, but since 1949, her home has been in the United States. Currently she lives in Orange County, California. Marjory pioneered the teaching of Chinese language in the Los Angeles public schools in 1963. She was also the first Chinese-born woman to receive degrees in both Music Therapy (BMus., Alverno College) and in Ethnomusicology (Ph.D. University of California, Los Angeles). Her MusM., degree from the University of Southern California, was in Music Education. Additionally, she specialized in Asian Philosophies and Aesthetics. After teaching in various educational institutions for over forty years, she retired from Arizona State University in 1989. Her articles have been published in China, Germany, and the USA; and she wrote the entries on Taoism (Daoism) in the six-volume encyclopedia of world belief systems, *A Treasury of Mystic Terms,* published in New Delhi in 1989. Marjory's current goals are to simplify her life, enjoy her family and friends, and to live in peace and harmony in the world.

Kathy Recupero (b. 1942) is originally from Los Angeles. The second of six children, she graduated from College of Holy Names, Oakland, California, with a major in mathematics, and worked at the Jet Propulsion Laboratory in Pasadena. She later became a stay-at-home mom and enjoyed raising her three children. In 1973, she and her husband started a consulting business in governmental relations. Actively seeking enrichment through cultural experiences, she and her husband were living in Kenmare, County Kerry, Ireland, for three months while this contribution was edited and finalized.

William (Bill) Reid (b. 1930) started work as an apprentice mechanic at the age of 14 in the coal mines. He moved with his family from Fife, Scotland, to Lancashire, England, in 1947, where he finished his seven-year apprenticeship. While working full time, he attended day and evening college courses, achieving graduate membership in The Institution of Mechanical Engineers. In October 1956, he immigrated to California with his wife and three-year old son, and was later blessed with a daughter. With his first California employer, he progressed from draftsperson to project engineer. In 1963 he was recruited as chief engineer of a manufacturing company, and in 1967, was appointed Vice President of Manufacturing and Engineering, a position he retained when his company was acquired by a Fortune 500 U.S. company. He became Vice President of Engineering when the firm later became a major division of a British conglomerate. Surviving bypass surgery at age 52 (and again at age 67), he retired at age 61. He and his wife designed their home in the High Sierras and created gardens for their two homes; he also shared skiing and fly fishing interests with his grandson and made movies and videos. In recent years, he helped his daughter with her business. Today, living in Fountain Valley with his wife of 576 years, his writing is an extension of scriptwriting and digital editing for his cinematography hobbies.

Joanne Simpson (b. 1935) from Duluth, Minnesota, moved to California in 1942. She graduated from Bell High School, where she sang leading roles in the school's musicals, earned speech, music and leadership awards, and was a class Ephebian scholar. A representative to Girls State of California, she was elected their Secretary of State in 1952. Awarded a full scholarship to Pepperdine College, she received a BA in Drama, Speech Arts, and English. Her General Secondary Credential was earned at Cal State Los Angeles in 1958.

She retired in 2000 after teaching for forty two years in junior and senior high school in Glendale, Walnut Creek, Orinda, and Buena Park, California. A former president of the Buena Park Teacher's Association, she is now a volunteer at the Crystal Cathedral, Garden Grove, and is a facilitator for their Divorce and Grief Recovery Group. She has a daughter, a son-in-law, and four grandchildren.

Marie Thompson is a contented British transplant, now living in California. Throughout her life, she has appreciated all aspects of the arts, along with a profound respect for the natural world. She endeavors to show within her short stories the extraordinary in the ordinary through her fascination with the everyday marvels of life around her. Her experience as an art buyer for a major advertising agency in London, a freelance film production assistant, and an analyst of children's art for a university in the United States has allowed access to many opportunities of interest. An eclectic list of hobbies includes skydiving, martial arts, theatre, crime scene investigation, and psychology ensured an expansion of herself. She is grateful to her daughter, Karen, whose poetry lifts her spirit, her son, Guy, who is able to capture the California light in his paintings, and her son, Scott, whose black and white photography captures many earth wonders. She excitedly awaits the talents of her young grandchildren to be revealed.

Phan Vũ (b. 1933) is from Thanh Hóa Province, Vietnam. As a schoolteacher, he taught French in Sóc Trăng,

Biên Hòa, and Nhà Bè high schools. He diligently carried out his military duty in the South Vietnam Army in 1962. After the fall of Saigon in April 1975, he was interned in Bà Tô re-education prison, then came to the United States in April 1993 under the Humanitarian Operation Program. He graduated from CSU Long Beach in 2000, majoring in English—Creative Writing. He is now a participant in the Huntington Beach Adult School Writing Workshop with Dr. Ross Winterowd. Phan Vũ's wife, Đính Lê, teaches high school French, and they live in Westminster, California. They have a daughter, Audrey, in Los Angeles, and a son Minh, in Fontana, San Bernardino County.

Edna Woolley (b. 1922) is from Muscatine, a small town on the banks of the Mississippi, in southeastern Iowa. After graduating from high school, Edna married and moved to Chicago. Her first child, a boy, was born there, and they moved to California when he was four. Seven years later, she added two girls to her family, and five years later another boy. She realized this was all she could handle. (With her background of eighteen siblings, it was all she wanted.) After a dissolution of marriage twenty-five years later, she studied music, acting, and writing at Goldenwest College in Huntington Beach, California, in addition to giving private voice instruction at the college for ten years. Later, she joined a group singing locally for entertainment. She then began to study writing, and now realizes her heart is in writing. Beginning with extended family genealogy, writing with the aid of historical records, she has now branched out to stories of immediate family, while the experiences are still fresh in her mind. With her unusual family background, she has a lot to write about.

Richard Wrate (b. 1931) In a world of Depression, a mother felt joy holding her first-born. The father searched for work with little success. Their address changed nineteen times in six years, and in a final effort to ease the burden, they moved once more. On an uncle's farm there were berries to pick and a garden to plant. This helped feed the large extended family of eleven. Two miles distant was a one room schoolhouse, where eleven Babcock family members and Richard wasted time under the tutelage of the Babcock's unqualified cousin. Little Dickie became the social outcast. December 7th, 1941, found the Wrate family moving to South Bend, Indiana, where their father made aircraft parts. The terrified boy was exposed to a thousand peering faces at the huge school, but an angel lifted him from F's to A's and B's. Miss Vivian Herring, a dedicated teacher, spent evenings tutoring the backward country boy. Although slowly dying from cancer; she found time to offer guidance. With high school and two years of college behind him, Richard joined the Navy, and later, in 1958, he graduated from Long Beach State. After four years with Moore Business Forms, he opened a mail order business, then retired forty years later. There was time to enjoy the family and his four grandchildren, with time to write, a garden to grow, and a wife of forty-six years to grow old with.

Breinigsville, PA USA
30 March 2011
258775BV00001B/147/P